Patient's Fight Against Cancer

Eula Youngblood

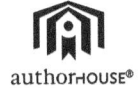

authorHOUSE®

AuthorHouse™
1663 Liberty Drive, Suite 200
Bloomington, IN 47403
www.authorhouse.com
Phone: 1-800-839-8640

First published by AuthorHouse   2/5/2008

ISBN: 978-1-4343-4579-0 (sc)

Library of Congress Control Number: 2007908082

Printed in the United States of America
Bloomington, Indiana

This book is printed on acid-free paper.

Cover design: Starlyn Kelly Youngblood

RESEACH CONTRIBUTIONS

1. Natural Health Solutions

2. Life Time Reports of Tung Hai Chlorella

3. Sun Chlorella

4. Cedar Sinai Cancer Research Center

5. ACCN and ACS Team

6. Massachusetts General Hospital Cancer Society

7. American Cancer Society

8. New York Magazine's Interview of 141 Cancer Patients

9. F C & A Medical Center, NY, NY

10. Sloan Caner Memorial Center, NY, NY

11. Anderson Medical Center Houston, Texas

12. Personal testimonies of relatives, neighbors and! friends

13. U.S. Oncology News

10% of all sales from this book will be donated to The American Cancer Society Research Fund and at their liberty; to assist hardship patients receive treatments.

RESEARCH TEAM FOR THIS PUBLICATION

- Kent Tracy Youngblood

- Starlyn Kelly Youngblood

- Dr. Miguel Pablo Medina M,D. (Oncologist; Kaiser Permanente Medical Clinic)

PROOF READING

Dr. Miguel Pablo Medina M.D. Kaiser Permanente

ALLITERATION STEPS TO SUCCESS

1. EDUCATE: The most important step towards defeating cancer is to learn all about it.

2. CONGREGATE: Get together with others to discuss your cancer concerns, perhaps in a group therapy setting,

3. PARTICIPATE: Volunteer to help others; cope with their fears, by discussing positive histories that you know of cancer treatment, and survivals.

4. ACTUATE: Develop plans of attack, something that you can do to prevent cancer; such as proper diet, non-smoking, or alcohol, and drug abuse, rest and exercise.

5. MEDICATE: Follow your primary care physician, and oncologist's medical plan. Keep a journal of medicines, and treatments.

6. ANNIAHLATE: By following the above steps, and diligently seeking medical help, together with cancer research, counseling, and following your doctor's advice, we may rid our society of this evil, and deadly disease.

CHAPTER ONE

My first day in the Chemotherapy treatment room was depressing. There were seven reclining chairs, with aside attached table for treatment equipment, and a swivel gooseneck television for the patients entertainment during the two and one half, to five hours of treatment required for each patient, depending on their type of cancer and treatment required for each stage of the disease.

As I entered the silent room that had two Registered nurses fluttering around the room in response to the bells ringing on various treatment pumps, letting them know that something needed to be done, with the intravenous pumps. I noticed that the patients were silent, or whispering softly to their relatives who'd come to cheer them.

All of the patients sat around with sad expressions on their faces. Their expressions were of fear, dread, and drained of life, with wrinkles covering their foreheads. I could see they had determined that the Grim Reaper had all of their names on his hit list., and was coming to collect his booty.

My thoughts were I could not spend more than six months in this depressing situation? Something had to be done to change their imaginary execution room, to something more positive. They needed a place where cancer patients can come together in a more positive attitude to fight this evil umsympathetic crab that reaches out to infect anyone within reach of its tentacles.

I knew instantly that several things were missing in the minds of those sad people. The missing things were hope, faith, charity, and education. We all have a tendency to fear those things that we don't understand. I had to somehow make my fellow suffering companions understand their affliction, and how they could arm themselves to fight back.

"That's it," I thought. "I'm a writer, and I'll write a book from the patient's viewpoint, explaining all about cancer, and how patients can help themselves. "Why not?" If what I'd say now got their attention that would be a feather in the win category.

"Hello everybody." I began. "My name is Eula Youngblood. I just had two feet of my ascending colon removed with cancer. This is the third time I've had to fight this evil creature off for trying to steal away my freedom. I will not allow it to take away my will to live. We must all hang together, and fight. We will prevail through it if we fight.

"Evil loves darkness, so we must attack the enemy in the dark corners where it lurks. It is difficult for the doctors to find this enemy sometimes; because of the sneaky way it lurks in the shadows of our bodies. So let's hang together, and fight this evil crab on his territory. We can win if we try."

"Organization, and education are the weapons that we need to gain a victory. So let's get together, and send that ugly crab cancer straight back to hell where it belongs."

A bent, saddened young mother of two young boys sat holding onto her husband's hand for support, stared up at me, and a ray of hope sparkled in her sad eyes.. To my right, a seniorly woman whose hairless head glistened in the: fluorescent lights, and her cute little ski-sloped nose kept dribbling watery clear snot, but she was the first to speak up:

"Cancer has spread to many of my organs, but I'm a fighter, and am willing to fight with you, if you'll teach me how."

And then the questions began:

Where were your Cancers before? " Someone in the corner asked."

"In 1968,1 had Cancer of the Uterus, which resulted in a hysterectomy, and oophorectomy, and in 1986,1 had a lumpectomy for breast cancer. Since this is 2007; I'm a 39 year survivor of uterine cancer, and a 21 year survivor of breast cancer. I figure if old age doesn't take me first, cancer will not take me out. You can't stop a stepper.

"How did you know that you had cancer each time? Another question was directed at me."

"In the sixties, when certain types of birth control was used, it was necessary that women have a Pap Smear every six months. When I went to have my biannual check-up, Voila! I had a class III Pap smear that resulted in a hysterectomy, and oopharectomy the next day. And then when I seemed to be having a nervous breakdown under job stress in 1986, my doctor insisted that I needed to take hormones, even though I'd been instructed not to take them. Within two months, my breast was leaking fluid, and the result was a pea-sized lump next to the nipple of the left breast, an urgent mammogram, and biopsy revealed a malignancy, which resulted in a lumpectomy."

"This last time was colon cancer. The paramedics took me urgently to the emergency room with a cancelled heartbeat. An urgent pacemaker was recommended, but my blood count was too low. I was given the necessary transfusion to withstand pacemaker surgery, and the doctors began looking for the cause for the blood count to drop so low."

"Several iron infusions were administered, but the count kept dropping. A stool culture showed no blood in the stools. Then a colonoscopy was performed, and a large tumor was found in the ascending colon, but the biopsy was benign. That was done in March of 2006, and in November of 1996, a doctor tried to remove the tumor without general anesthesia, since I have COPD, and Congestive heart failure, but the mass was too large for his instruments."

"December 7, 2006, a laparotomy was done, and the tumor that had previously read negative on two occasions was found to be malignant, class II. The invasion had not included the lymph nodes, nor the liver, but chemotherapy was recommended since this was the third time my body had been invaded, and cancer is extremely secretive., and cells can hide in places that we least expect."

"I'll write a book," I said. "That will teach you what you need to know to arm yourselves. I hope it will be distributed to all cancer patients everywhere, and possibly those people who might be candidates to become a cancer patient in the future."

Another middle-aged woman spoke up, and her questions were so pessimistic.

"This disease is so debilitating. When you hear it's name, you know that your days are numbered."

"Oh ye of little faith." I quoted the Holy Scriptures. If we give up, the fight is lost. So often wives tales binds us to believe that if we have a hysterectomy, our sex lives are over, or by having a breast surgery, we are only half a woman, and men feel that if they have prostate surgery, their masculine lives have been terminated. These stories are not necessarily true.

If your mates are telling you this, there was not much *love* in the union anyway, or they are justifying an extra marital affair they are having, or plan to have soon.

My best friend, a lovely woman with a gorgeous figure, talked me through my breast cancer ordeal, allowing me to think that she had her lumpectomy months before my discovery. She's been dead for twelve years now, after turning down the simple treatment that could've saved her life. Her cancer spread throughout her body, raging like an uncontrollable forest fire, and the doctors could not save her. She lost her fight, because she did not want to lose her beautiful figure. What good is that kind of pride?

Another of my friend's husband, who'd just been diagnosed with prostate cancer, declared that he would not allow the doctors to mess around with his "family jewels". At forty-six, he left behind his lovely wife, and two beautiful daughters, when his pridefulness allowed the cancer to spread through his body.

My niece, who'd suffered for years with chromes disease, diagnosed herself, when she discovered a lump in her breast. She convinced herself that the lump was a new symptom of her current problem, and would go away eventually if she'd leave it alone. She suffered horribly before she passed away with metastasized cancer two years ago.

In 1990, one of my older brothers thought that the blood he found in his shorts, and stool, was hemorrhoids, and he bought suppositories to treat himself. He went to the doctor only after the problem had become painful, and he'd lost a lot of weight. He also died a very painful death, about a year after he'd discovered his problem.

The point that I'm trying to convey here is: don't start practicing medicine without a license. Allow your doctors to do the job he, or she was trained for years to do. And what good is it to save a few dollars, and your pride, if you are going to lose your life?

Be aware of industrial cover-ups!

Watch out for this activity. Always seek a second opinion away from your company's paid physicians.

Another of my brothers, who'd worked for an eastern steel mill for more than thirty years, was exposed to asbestos, and other chemicals. The company obviously paid the doctors at the veteran's clinic under the table, who used the band-aid method of treatment, when my brother started to exhibit symptoms that something was wrong.

My brother's constant bleeding from the nose, and gums; was treated with strange mouthwashes, and cauterization. His bloated abdomen, was treated with heavy doses of fiber. He had a number of other symptoms that his younger brother suggested he should seek advice from a private doctor, but he trusted the V. A. Doctors. His postmortem examination showed that he died from misothelioma, leukemia, and a multiple myoloma.

The trustees for the company are paying my late brother's relatives enough money to pay for a lunch at Jack-in-the-box, each month. My husband was also caught up in a huge chemical cover-up at Rockwell International. He was hospitalized in 1960 with Fever of Undetermined

Origin, and after two weeks of test, it was found that he had radiation exposure.

He also suffered a collapsed lung, several years later, and developed a chronic, but mild cough. The company's repeated test showed nothing wrong with him, but after a number of his ex-coworkers died with numerous types of cancer, he decided to join the research team at Cal. State, Irvine. And there, they found *a* prostate cancer lesion hidden far back on the prostate. He had surgery, and is doing fine except his cough. The Environmental Protection Agency has been investigating the company's cover-up, and a number of cancer victims have been compensated.

QUICK CURE CLAIMS

Beware of the "Sharks" who advertise medicines of cure that have never been proven. These people are out there to get your hard earned dollars through the sale of their literature, or their "Placebo, sugar pills. On June 1, 2007 at 9:00 pm, the television program 20/20 interviewed the CEO of a drug manufacturing firm called Manutech.

The CEO stated publicly that they never claimed that the drug they'd developed, and named 'Hope in a Bottle," was never stated to be able to cure cancer, but it was proven that the sales representatives are telling their customers that the drug is a sure cure.

A young college girl, whose father died of a brain tumor, that was the same as the girl now have stands by the "Hope-in-a-Bottle" sugar drug, and she refuses to have radiation, or chemotherapy to shrink her brain tumor . During a recent MRI, it was found that the small fist sized tumor, has had no size change.

We are all intelligent enough to know that when our cars have an engine knock, or is running hot, we'd better seek a mechanic quickly to avoid an expensive engine repair so, why is it not possible for many of us to recognize the warnings our body's gives to us also, and quickly seek medical help?

In some cases, cancer does not send us a warning that we can recognize as danger signals. That is why it is so important for us to get annual check-ups. Regular breast exams at home, or in your doctor's office, a regular colonoscopy, and other diagnostics are just as important.. Your physician has spent numerous years after high school, studying the human body, and I'm sure they know more than we do., or they'll refer us to a doctor in a specialized field who does.

Learn to read your Bible, and depend on the promises there in, that God made to you, such as is found in 1 Corinthians 10:13 "There hath no temptation taken you, but such as is common to man: But God is faithful, who will not permit you to be tempted, above that ye are able, but will with the temptation also make a way to escape, that ye may be able to bear it. Or, as found in St. Luke 8:48, and 17:19, "Thy faith hath healed thee." And, "If you will have the faith of a mustard seed, you can move mountains."

Remind God often of His promises He's made to you when you pray, and believe in them, and in yourself.

Chapter Two

EDUCATION

Cancer is the name used to describe a broad group of diseases, which have certain common characteristics. Most cells in the body grow, and reproduce in an orderly manner, as dictated by the body's genetic information. A cancer cell does not follow the same genetic direction that Normal body cells do,

Cancer cells grow at an uncontrolled rate, taking over, or causing the death of, or replacing normal cells as they grow inside the body. As cancer progresses, cells are often sent through the circulatory system to start growth in other parts of the body. When this occurs, this is called metastasis.

The term tumor, means literally, "a growth". A tumor may be either malignant, (cancerous), or benign,)not cancerous). A benign tumor commonly grows within a self produced capsule, and does not evade surrounding tissue (although it can cause problems by pressing on the surrounding tissue, nor does it spread itself throughout the body. Malignant tissue may grow out of control, and quite commonly spread.

There are over 2000 types of cancer that have been identified by pathologist, (the physicians who studies the body's tissue.) Despite the large number, there are three basic categories of cancer: CARCINOMA (cancer of the cells known as epithelium cells that finds organs, and serve many purposes, including production of mucous, and protection). SARCOMA (cancer of the bones, and muscle tissue's) and fluid cancers, (LEUKEMIA, is one example of a fluid cancer) some cancers may fall into more than one category.

WARNING SIGNS

_Often the patient is the first to suspect cancer. This is why it is important to learn cancer's seven warning signs:
1. **Change in bowel, and/or bladder habits**
2. **A sore that does not heal**
3. **Unusual bleeding, or discharge**
4. **Thickening, or lumps in the breast, or elsewhere.**
5. **Indigestion, or difficulty in swallowing.**
6. **Obvious change in warts, or moles.**
7. **A nagging cough or horseness.**

Since the chances of cure are grater for the cancer discovered at an early stage, you should learn to perform the important self-examinations. If you are a woman, you (or mate) should learn to perform the breast self-examinations, to detect suspicious lumps as early as possible. If you are a man, many physicians recommend testicle self-examinations for testicular cancer.

DIAGNOSIS

If you suspect you may have cancer, do not delay in seeing a physician, following a physical examination of the doctor suspects possible abnormal growth, he or she may order a series of tests, including X-ray exam (for example, tomograms or CAT SCANS which are X-rays utilizing an in-depth technique), nuclear medicine scans (liver scans-spleen scan, thyroid scan, ultrasound examination, cytology test (examination of body cells such as is done in a Pap Smear, and a group of laboratory evaluations.

The doctor may also order a biopsy (microscopic examination of a tissue sample) to determine the cell type of the suspected growth and whether it is benign or malignant.

Your physician may also refer you to a specialist in the area of your suspected cancer. This may be an oncologist (cancer specialist cancer surgeon, radiation therapist, hematologist specialist (specialist in blood disease) or a number of other specialized physicians. These physicians are specially trained to deal with diagnosis and treatment of your cancer.

There are many ways of treating cancer. Many treatment programs called protocols have been developed that have been most effective in certain types of disease. Cancer therapy often includes surgery to remove the cancer, to clear obstructions of vital passageways caused by the cancer, or to cut nerve paths sending pain messages to your brain; chemotherapy (use of powerful drugs to kill cancer cells, or a number of other newly developed techniques. Often, combinations of the above therapies are used.

Surgery is the most common method of dealing with tumors that develop into tumors. If cancer is contained on one area, surgery can sometimes completely eliminate it. New surgery techniques are continually expanding the race of tumors that can be safely removed. Furthermore, if the surgeon is only able to remove; a part of the tumor, the reduced tumor can often be controlled with eradiation, or chemotherapy.

More precise surgical techniques mean that surgery study are often less disfiguring than in the past. In addition, new developments in skin grafting make it possible to begin reconstructive work on patients-for instance, those with cancer of the head and neck-simultaneously with the cancer surgery. Sometimes surgery is performed on the patient, even though it is known that surgery will not cure the cancer. The removal of the tumor may simply make the patient more comfortable. In other cases, nerve pathways to the pain centers, may be cut. Certain non-cancerous growths may be removed, because they are a kind of growth that may develop into cancer.

Chemotherapy, the treatment of cancer with drugs, has gradually become much more significant. More than 12 kinds of cancer can now be effectively treated by chemotherapy alone. However, cancer drugs are most often used as an adjuvant that is as a backup to primary treatment such as surgery.

Once surgery has reduced a cancer, chemotherapy can most often eliminate it. Chemotherapy has proved effective against certain forms of cancer that used to be almost always fatal, particularly Hodgkin's disease, acute lymphocytic leukemia, (blood disease of children), and cancer of the testes, (the male sex gland).

Most cancer drugs attack any fast-reproducing cells in the body. Whether they are cancerous or not, producing some of the well-known side effects of chemotherapy.

Destruction of Normal cells that reproduce frequently such as those in the digestive track, the hair follicles, and the bone morrow, can lead to nausea, hair loss, and lowered red blood cell count. Usually several drugs are administered in combination, if the cancer does not respond, or a resistance to a drug develops, another combination may be attempted. Radiation destroys the ability of cells to divide. Cancer cells are far more susceptible to radiation than normal cells, although not all cells respond to radiation. Like surgery, radiation therapy is a localized treatment, directed at a particular cancer site. Radiation treatment may also involve directly implanting into tumor a radioactive pellet that destroys from within. Radiation can be used before surgery to reduce a tumor to operable size, and frequently, a patient receives radiation after surgery to destroy any cancer cells that might remain near the cancer site, Some tumors can be treated by radiation alone. Radiation can be especially useful in cancers for which surgery will impair basic bodily functions. For example, surgery for cancer of the testes may leave the patient impotent, while radiation treatment avoids this. Radiation treatment of cancer of the larynx preserves the voice box, and in the case; of breast cancer, radiation can prevent the disfiguring effects of surgery. However, in these forms of cancer, surgery may often be necessary, Radiation therapy is being continually refined. Drugs have been discovered that make cancer cells more sensitive to radiation. Different forms of radiation are being tested on resistant cancers. In addition, radiation today can be directed more precisely, and stronger forms with little harm to overlying tissue.

However, there are still side effects including loss of appetite, nausea, and hair loss. It is not certain how dangerous it is to be treated with radiation, which is itself a carcinogen. However, it is believed that a cancer in the body is far more threatening, than the future effects of radiation therapy.

IMMUNOTHERAPY, is to enable the patient's own body to produce substances that resist the growth of cancer. The basis of immunotherapy, while still being experimental,. Is the theory that cancer develops when for some reason, the body fails to destroy abnormal cells. So far, immunotherapy is still in the experimental stage.

Interferon is a natural substance produced by the body to resist viruses. In the laboratory interferon has been observed to prevent cancer cells from multiplying. Yet so far, interferon has been very costly to produce artificially, and in tests it has not been as effective as standard treatment. It is likely that in the future, strengthening the body's defenses will become an important weapon against cancer.

Heat Therapy or hypothermia, now being used experimentally, may soon become standard treatment for some kinds of cancer. Tumors have been shown to shrink when their temperature is raised. The circulation inside tumors is much more sluggish than in normal tissue-thus a tumor can usually endure far less heat.

Temperatures tolerable to normal cells can be deadly to cancers. Heat therapy is largely painless. An instrument called a magnetrode can deliver heat to inner portions of the body without harming overlying tissue. However, not all patients can be treated with hypothermia, the location of the tumor or the weakened health of the patient may rule out heat therapy. At this point, heat therapy has been most effective when used in combination with radiation or chemotherapy.

Laetrile is an extract of apricot pits that some have proclaimed is a cure for cancer. This substance has been branded because it has been shown to be of no value against cancer in laboratory animals and has yet to be adequately tested in humans. Most patients who have shown a response to lact rile have also received conventional cancer therapy

Sometimes a patient or his family will seek unorthodox methods of cancer treatment such as laetrile. The medical community is actively researching all known methods of treating cancer and carefully evaluating those that look most promising. Many treatments are slow, and often have severe side effects.

The harm done by quack practitioners is that they prevent a patient from seeking effective treatment until it is too late for any treatment to be of use. The best advice is to trust a physician to treat cancer and not waste time, money, and hope on an unproven unlicensed quack cure.

There are many places to get cancer treatment. Most cancers can be effectively treated by a well-equipped, and staffed community hospital. There are, however a number of large cancer centers throughout the country where specialized protocols are available. Often diagnosis and or treatment is initiated at a real center, and then continued in the community by an oncologist and or family physician.

If you need information, or referrals to cancer hotlines or the American Cancer Society and valuable resources. In the event you wish a second opinion about your case, either recourse, or your personal physician should assist you in getting another evaluation

THOSE AT RISK

Who develops cancer? This is a question that is very difficult, if not impossible to answer. There are, however, certain risk factors that increase the possibility that you may develop cancer in your lifetime. Among these are age. As a rule, the older you are, the higher your risk of getting cancer. In some cases family history for example, if your mother or sister had breast cancer, your risk of developing breast cancer is increased; and environmental and other factors.

The rapid increase in cancer rages during this century has been blamed, to a large part, on the environment. Polluted air and water, food additives and colorings, changes. In diet from "natural", to "processed" foods all have been implicated as possible causes. Cigarette smoking has been shown to be a cause of lung and other related cancers. If you wish to reduce your risk of getting cancer it is important to control the factors that you can control-obviously one person alone cannot clean the environment. However, you can stop smoking.

PROGNOSTIC FACTORS

If you do develop cancer, there are a number of prognostic factors (factors that predict length of survival) that are important. Most important are the stage and the type of the disease. The earlier the stage of the disease, that of the disease, that is, the sooner it is diagnosed, the better the prognosis will be. The type of tumor also makes a major difference, since different tumors respond differently to treatment.

Furthermore, within a specific organ there are different cell types of cancer that can occur. For example, all lung cancers are not the same type of cells. Often these types are important in determining both response to therapy, and prognosis. Your age and overall physical condition are also important in determining your ability to win the fight over cancer.

Cancer should no longer be considered the dreaded scourge that it was thought to be 20 years ago. It is not always fatal and is in many instances curable. The keys to living today should be to avoid cancer-causing materials, (for example. Cigarettes), to consult your physician regularly (and discuss possible increased risk factors), and to perform regularly the important self-examination procedures that your doctor suggests. Early detection is of extreme importance and you are the best source of early detection.

TYPES OF CANCER

Bladder cancer: This is the most common cancer of the urinary tract. It occurs most often between the ages of 50 and 70, and is the fourth leading cause of cancer deaths among men. Four times as many men as women are afflicted.

Bladder cancer has been connected with exposure to a number of carcinogens. This may be because the urinary tract comes into contact with so many foreign substances because of its excretory function. For many years, it has been known that those who work with aniline dyes have a high incidence of cancer of the bladder.

Bladder cancer is also associated with tar from tobacco smoke and with schistosomia infestation, a tropical parasite. Blood in the urine is usually the first symptom of bladder cancer, in addition, urination may be difficult, painful, and frequent. The appearance of blood in the urine may be intermittent, and sometimes if this symptom disappears a doctor is not consulted. However, anyone with blood in the urine should consult a doctor since in early stages this disease is highly curable, and treatment is far more difficult later on. If your doctor feels the symptoms suggests bladder cancer, he or she may order a cystoscopy. Under local anesthesia a lighted tube called a cystoscope is passed into the urinary tract through the urethra (the passageway from the bladder to the outside), through which the interior of the bladder can be examined. This instrument can even take a biopsy (removal of a small piece of tissue for analysis) of a suspicious growth.

Treatment of bladder cancer depends on how far advanced the disease is. A small tumor can sometimes be completely removed by a cystoscope. More advanced cases are treated by surgery^ or radiation or a combination of the two.

BONE CANCER: This is a rare form of cancer most common in children between the ages of five and 15. Predisposing factors to bone cancer are bone diseases, bone fractures, and exposure to radiation. Bone cancer begins with a sarcoma, the name for a tumor that develops in muscle, bone or cartilage (the elastic tissue of the ends of bones).

Bone cancer usually develops first in the arms or legs. Pain, swelling, or brittle of bone may be its symptoms. X-ray can often tell whether the bone is cancerous. and if the disease has spread. If cancer is indicated, and orthopedic surgeon should perform a biopsy. Bone cancer is usually treated by a combination of surgery, radiation, and chemotherapy.

BRAIN CANCER Any tumor in the brain, whether cancerous or not, is very dangerous. Because the brain occupies an enclosed space within the skull, even a small tumor that weighs only a fifth of a pound can cause crowding sufficient to bring on death. Brain cancer is most often the result of metastasis from other cancer sites, particularly the breast, lung, and skin.

Symptoms of brain cancer are of two kinds. Increased pressure in the skull can cause seizures, headaches, nausea, forgetfulness, and personality changes. However, symptoms may also arise in the part of the body controlled by the affected area in the brain. For instance coordination, vision, or strength of limbs may be affected. In the past, brain tumors have not responded we'll to the development of the disease. Recently, however diagnostic techniques have improved.

The CAT (computerized axial tomography) scanner produces a three-dimensional image of the brain that can clearly determine the size and location of a tumor. By using a CAT scanner, doctors are also able to monitor carefully the progress of any treatment.

Surgery is the primary treatment for brain cancer when the disease has not spread throughout the body. Surgery in the brain is a delicate procedure; often a tumor deep in the brain cannot be totally removed without risking impairment of body function. however, new techniques in brain surgery sometimes with the use of a microscope-permit treatment of tumors once considered inoperable. Radiation or chemotherapy will often follow surgery through the sensitivity of brain tissue demands that these be administered cautiously. Steroid drugs will often be given to reduce the dangerous swelling that a tumor can produce.

Breast Cancer; About one woman in 13 will develop breast cancer at some time in her life. It is the leading cause of cancer death in women, and the leading cause of all death in women between the ages of 40 and 44. The high risk group includes women over 35, women who have never had children or who have had a child for the first time after the age of 30, and women who began menstruation early or who experienced late menopause. Breast cancer also occurs more frequently in chemical workers, women with a family history of this disease, and women who have already had breast cancer.

Self Examination of the breast can often lead to early detection. All women particularly those in the high risk category should perform these examinations monthly at the end of the menstrual period. Approximately 90 percent of all breast cancers are first discovered by self-examination.

THE RECOMMENDED TECHNIQUE FOR BREAST SELF-EXAMINATION IS AS FOLLOWS:

1. In the shower, keep one hand overhead and examine each breast with opposite hand, wet, or soapy skin may make it easier to feel lumps.

2. Lying in bed, place a pillow under one shoulder, to evaluate and flatten breast, Examine each breast, with the opposite hand, first with arm under head and again with arm at side.

3. In front of a mirror stand with hands resting on hips. Examine breast for swelling, dimpling, bulges, and changes in skin.

4. Make rotary motions-with flat pads, hot tips, of fingers-in concentric circles inward toward nipple. Feel for knots, lumps, or indentations. Be sure to include the armpit area.

5. In front of mirror, examine breasts for changes with arms extended overhead. This position highlights bulges, and indentations that may indicate a lump.

6. Squeeze nipples gently to inspect for any discharge, Report any suspicious findings to your doctor.

If a lump is discovered in the breast, your doctor will probably order an X-ray of the breast, known as a mammogram. The doctor may also recommend a thermo gram, which can detect growths by measuring body heat. This test is based on the premise that new growths may generate more heat 1han the surrounding tissue. However, thermograph is not as accurate as mammography and should be used only to augment mammogram.

The doctor may also take a biopsy (the tissue sample) of the lump to test for the presence of cancer is indicated, surgery will probably be performed. Women with breast cancer often dread surgery because of the disfigurement that can result, however, today surgery for a breast tumor is often less extensive than in the past. At one time all breast cancer patients received a radical mastectomy, or removal of the breast, underlying chest muscles, and lymph glands in the armpit. Now it is known that in many cases the removal of the breast, or even the tumor alone, may be equally effective. In addition, there are techniques for reconstruction of the breast after surgery and re validation of muscles tone in an arm that has been weakened by surgery

In some cases, radiation therapy will be used after surgery to destroy any remaining cancer cells.

Cancer of the Colon: About 40,000 Americans die every year of cancer of the colon, and rectum. About half of all cases of cancer of the colon can be cured by surgery, and early detection can greatly improve this percentage. A simple test for blood in the stool can indicate whether further test should be made for the presence of this cancer.

Everyone over 40, or with chronic digestive problems, should have this test regularly. Chance of cure is twice as likely if the disease is discovered before symptoms occur.

Symptoms of cancer of the colon include a change in stools or in bowel movement, bleeding from the rectum, pencil thin stools, and abdominal discomfort not eased by bowel movement. If you have any of these symptoms your doctor will probably perform a rectal exam, (inserting a finger into the rectum). To search for unusual growths. If further examination is necessary, the doctor may introduce a sigmoidoscope (a lighted tube) into the colon through the anus, the opening end of the intestine.

This instrument permits examination of the inside of the colon and can also take a biopsy of suspicious growths. Sometimes a cancerous polyp is removed by a similar instrument, because such polyps may sometimes develop into cancer.

Surgery is the usual treatment for cancer of the colon. If the cancer is near to or in the rectum, the surgeon may remove all the rectum and create an artificial rectum, or colostomy, in the lower abdominal wall. A colostomy is usually covered with a bag to collect waste material.

CANCER OF THE CERVIX: The cervix is the lower part of the uterus, or womb, that extends into the vagina. Cancer of the cervix is the second most common cancer among American women. The death rate from this disease has decreased 50 percent over the last 50 years, largely as a result of early diagnosis.

Early cervical cancer has no symptoms but can be detected by a Pap Smear.

A pap smear is performed routinely in a doctor's office by scraping the surface of the cervix. The collected material is then tested for indications of cancer. Today two out of three cases of cervical cancer are detected by a Pap smear before they display symptoms.

Cervical cancer has a higher incidence among black women and poor women. This cancer also occurs more frequently among women who were sexually active early with many partners and among those with genital herpes.

If a Pap smear indicates the possibility of cervical cancer, a biopsy of the affected area will probably be performed. Treatment depends on how far the disease had advanced; early forms are almost always curable by surgical removal of the cervix and uterus called a hysterectomy, If a patient still hopes to bear children, and the cancer is in an early stage, sometimes this surgery can be put off until after children have been born. However, this is possible only if the disease does not seem to be progressing, and the cancer must be monitored carefully during this phase. Eventually the uterus should be removed. More advanced forms of the disease are treated with radiation as well as surgery.

LEUKEMIA this is a disease of the bone morrow, the site of blood cell production. Blood cells called platelets control clotting, white blood cells fight infecting; and red blood cells carry oxygen throughout the body. The symptoms of leukemia result from the impairment of these functions.

Leukemia is the most common form of cancer in children. In recent years, the outlook has improved dramatically for children suffering from leukemia. Twenty years ago nearly all children diagnosed as having leukemia died. Today close to 50 percent are cured-and the lives of many more are prolonged.

More than half the people diagnosed as having leukemia first consult a doctor with complaints of being very tired a result of low red blood cells count. Other symptoms are easy bruising, bleeding from the gums, blood in the stool, fever, and frequent infections. The spleen and lymph glands are usually enlarged.

A diagnosis of leukemia should be made by a cancer specialist. The doctor will probably insert a needle into the hipbone to withdraw bone marrow cells that will be tested for the presence of cancer.

Leukemia is often treated first with intensive chemotherapy to kill all cancer cells in the body. The patient may become even sicker during treatment because of the large dosages of cancer fighting drugs. After this initial treatment faze, radiation and additional drugs may be administered to be sure all of the disease has disappeared.

LIVER CANCER: Liver cancer usually results from the spread of cancer cells from another site in the body. However, cancer that originates in the liver can sometimes be traced to environmental carcinogens. It is known that any one who has worked with vinyl chloride, a chemical used in plastics manufacture has a higher risk of this disease. It also appears that cirrhosis of the liver, a disease in which normal liver cells are replaced by fibrous tissue, may cause an individual to be more susceptible to cancer of the liver. Symptoms of liver cancer are difficult to identify. Often they resemble the sign of a peptic ulcer-aching or burning pain in the upper abdomen, nausea, and vomiting. A swollen or hardened liver often indicates to the doctor the need for further testing. in the rare cases in which this cancer is diagnosed early ,and is confined to the liver, it can be treated surgically, but most often the prognosis is not good.

LUNG CANCER: Cigarette smoking is generally accepted, as the major cause of lung cancer. Lung cancer is the leading cause of cancer death in men, although in recent years the incidence of lung cancer in women is growing, probably as a result of increasing numbers of women who smoke, in addition, lung cancer is also increasing among nonsmokers. This may be due to improved diagnostic techniques (many lung tumors were once diagnosed as tuberculosis), as well as to increased environmental pollution.

If you smoke and are over 45, or have a family history of this disease, you should be on the look out for symptoms, since the early signs can be very mild, a persistent cough or lingering respiratory discomfort.

Later, coughing will increase as will chest pain and shortness of breath. The patient may also cough up blood.

A cancerous tumor in the lung is usually removed by surgery. To eliminate the entire tumor, it may be necessary to remove an entire lobe of the lung. Because lung cancers are usually not detected until they are well advanced, surgery alone may not be able to eliminate them, and radiation and chemotherapy will be used in combination with surgery.

In recent years the deadliest form of lung cancer, small-cell carcinoma has yielded to a net drug therapy that has produced significant remission in some patients.

LYMPHOMA: This cancer attacks the lymphatic system, particularly the lymph nodes and the spleen; These organs manufacture lymphocytes, cells that protect the body against infection.

The first symptoms of lymphoma are usually a swollen spleen or swollen lymph glands in the neck, armpit, or groin, (the juncture between the lower abdomen and the inner thigh). Fever and bad sweating are later symptoms. If these symptoms persist a doctor should be consulted. If the doctor suspect's cancer, he or she will probably order a biopsy tissue sample of that enlarged organ.

There are two major forms of lymphoma: Hodgkin's disease and non-Hodgkin's lymphoma. In recent years there have been dramatic strides in the treatment of Hodgkin's disease. In early stages, radiation alone can be very effective. Later in the development of the disease, more extensive radiation may be required, or a combination of radiation, and chemotherapy treatment of non-Hodgkin's lymphoma is much the same as that of Hodgkin's, but far fewer patients are cured. This form of the disease is usually discovered too late for treatment.

CANCER OF THE OVARY: This is the most dangerous form of cancer of the female reproductive organs, because it is so difficult to diagnose in its early stages. Women over 50 have a higher incidence of the disease, as do childless women and those with a family history of ovarian cancer.

Symptoms may include pelvic discomfort, constipation, abdominal swelling, and irregular menstruation. Often a diagnosis cannot be made without an exploratory operation known as a laparoscope's, during which the disease can be evaluated and, in some cases, treated.

In ovarian cancer usually both ovaries and the uterus are surgically removed, although sometimes it is possible to remove only one ovary. After surgery, radiation or chemotherapy may be administered.

PROSTATECANCER: After lung cancer, this is the most common cancer among men. Black Americans have a higher incidence of prostate cancer than any other group in the world. In general, it is more common in men over 55. Prostate cancer can develop very slowly and it often produces no symptoms until the disease is far advanced. Sometimes a routine examination turns up a lump in the prostate, which will prove to be cancerous in about 50 percent of the cases. Prostate examinations should be included in medical checkups of all men over 50.

When symptoms occur, they are usually the result of an enlarge prostate, the male gland that lies at the base of the bladder. The enlargement causes difficult urination, or blood in the urine. Prostate cancer often spread to the bones and patients may complain of bone pain before they show any other symptoms.

In the small percentage of cases, in which prostate cancer is discovered before it has begin to spread, the cancer can be removed by surgery or radiation. Since surgery may cause the patient to become impotent and unable to control urine flow, radiation is the preferred treatment for small tumors. When the disease has spread usually only its symptoms are treated as they occur. Often a patient can live a long time with this form of treatment.

SKIN CANCER: About 300,000 cases of skin cancer are discovered every year. Its incidence increases every year, particularly among women, perhaps because people currently are getting more exposure to sunlight. The ultra violet rays of the sun are a major cause of skin cancer. Fair-skinned people, lacking in a protective substance in the skin called melanin, are more susceptible to the effects of these rays than are dark-skinned people.

Skin cancer can also result from prolonged exposure to certain chemicals such as arsenic compounds, Burn scars and skin diseases sometimes develop into cancer.

Most skin cancers are highly treatable. Some can be removed in a doctor's office or in an outpatient clinic. But since some forms of these cancers can spread throughout the body, it is important that they be treated early.

The most dangerous skin cancer the malignant melanoma, can metastasize, throughout the body, it is important that they be treated early. The most dangerous skin cancer, the malignant melanoma, can metastasize through the lymph glands.

Melanomas usually develop from moles, though only about one mole in a million ever becomes a melanoma.

Symptoms of skin cancer are a chance in the surface of the skin, wounds that do not heal, and a sudden major change in a wart, mole, or birthmark, All such suspicious signs should be examined by a doctor.

Skin cancer is an unusual form of cancer in that it can be prevented easily. Fair-skinned people and anyone with a family history of skin cancer should avoid exposure to the sun. Additionally, everyone who spends time in the sun should apply a protective sunscreen to exposed portions of the body. It is important to remember that the use of certain drugs, such as barbiturates, antibiotics, and birth control pills, can increase the sensitive itself the skin, in addition, children with their more sensitive skin should be protected against the sun.

STOMACH CANCER: Stomach cancer has decreased 50 percent in the last 2 years. A change in diet may account for this. Stomach cancer is more common in men than women and usually occurs between the ages of 50 and 70. The high-risk group includes those with a history of pernicious anemia or alcoholism, arid persons with a diet rich in smoked, pickled or salted foods.

Symptoms of stomach cancer are similar to those of peptic ulcer (heartburn and Abdominal discomfort, making diagnosis more difficult). It may not be until the disease is well advanced that identifying symptoms of a bloody stool or vomit appear. To find a tumor a doctor will take a special X-ray that involves swallowing barium, a substance that coats the lining of the stomach so that it will show up on a photography.

If a tumor is indicated, a flexible tube known as an endoscopes may be inserted down the throat into the stomach to examine the tumor more closely and perhaps take a biopsy of it.

Surgery is the most effective treatment of this disease, but only about 10 percent of victims survive more than five years after diagnosis. Surgery is most useful when the tumor has not begun to spread. Sometimes it is necessary to remove all or part of the stomach. After such surgery, a patient will have to consume a low-bulk, high -protein diet.

CANCER OF THE UTERUS: This disease is most common in women over 50, especially susceptible are women who have never born children, and those who are obese, diabetic, or suffer from high blood pressure. Some women who have taken the female hormone estrogen to control symptoms of menopause are also in the high risk group.

Vaginal bleeding after menopause is the most common symptom of uterine cancer. If a Pap smear shows no abnormalities, then minor surgery, known as a dilation and curettage, may be performed. This involves scraping the interior walls of the uterus in order to examine the tissue for the presence of cancer.

If cancer is indicated, a hysterectomy *surgical removal of he uterus and the ovaries, is usually performed, although hormones may be an effective treatment against this form of cancer. Cancer of the uterus is harder to detect than that of the cervix, it is often discovered after it is too advanced for successful treatment.

CANCER OF THE VAGINA: Once a disease confined to women over 50, in recent years cancer of the vagina has also begun to appear in some women between the ages of 17 and 20. The mothers of most of these young women took artificial estrogens during pregnancy, particularly the drug DBS (diethylstilbestrol, in order to prevent miscarriage).

Any woman whose mother took artificial estrogens during pregnancy should have a Pap smear twice a year. Symptoms of vaginal cancer include vaginal pain and bleeding. The disease is usually treated by radiation.

CHAPTER THREE

Although we've learned a lot about various types of cancer, I feel that there is never too much knowledge for us to absorb if we intend to defeat a disease called cancer. Therefore, like in the Holy 'scriptures, the writers have a tendency to repeat those laws, or rules that pertain to the way God wants us to govern our lives, and train our young people.

I feel that the more you understand about cancer, the better your chances of defeating it. Therefore, I will redefine types of cancer, and its symptoms, and treatments often to acquaint you with the battle that lies ahead. And as my research finds information that I feel will benefit us in our fight, I will fill that new information in.

<u>SOME CANCERS. AND ITS TREATMENT:</u>

BONE CANCER:

Bones make up a person's skeleton and provide a strong frame for muscles to work against. Bones also protect the body's vital organs. Bone tissue changes constantly. Cancers of the bones usually start in another location and spread to the bone (metastases). Cancers that start in the bone are quite rare.

The most common type of bone cancer is multiple mycelia,, which starts in the cells that make up bone marrow. Marrow is the soft fleshy material in the center of the bone. This type of bone cancer is seen mostly in older people.

The second highest number of bone cancer is osteosarcoma, which causes pain and swelling. While these tumors can start any where in the body they usually show up in or around the knee. Often they spread to the lungs. Rarely seen in young people 10 to 20 years of age, these tumors can, however, occur at any age.

There are several other types of bone cancer, including those affecting cartilage tissue, arms and legs. Often, bones become cancerous because the disease present in another part of the body has spread Most likely to spread are breast, lung, prostate, kidney and thyroid cancers.

SYMPTOMS:

Pain and swelling of bones and joints is usually the primary sign of the disease. Sometimes, fractures caused by weakened bones are also an indication.

DIAGNOSIS

Methods for detecting bone cancer depend on the type and stage of the disease. Options include:

- Biopsy: A small amount of tissue is taken from the bone and examined under the microscope for cancer cells.

- X-rays and bone scans: Standard X-rays and computed topography (CT) and magnetic resonance imaging (MRI) images can help find the size and exact location of the tumor

- Surgery: The tumor is removed from the affected area of the body most often the limbs . Today, amputation is very rarely done because of newer and more effective surgical methods are now used.

- Chemotherapy and/or radiation. Anti-cancer drugs may be given at some point in the treatment process as well as high-energy X-rays to destroy or shrink cancerous tissue.

BREST CANCER TRERATMENT, AND PROCEDURES: NON SURGICAL TREATMENTS:

- Chemotherapy

- Radiation Therapy

- Hormone Therapy

- Integrative Medicine

- Women's Health

- Physical Therapy for lymph edema SURGICAL TREATMENTS:

- Auxiliary Node Dissection

- Lumpectomy/Segmental Mastectomy

- Radical Mastectomy

- Modified Radical Mastectomy

- Skin-Sparing Mastectomy

- Sentinel (Blue) Node Biopsy

- Breast Plastic and Reconstructive Surgery

- Post-surgical Treatment PREPARING FOR YOUR PRECEDURE

- Bilateral Screening Mammogram/ bilateral Diagnostic

- Ultrasound

- Stereo tactic Breast Biopsy

- Needle Localized Breast Biopsy

- Surgical Biopsy CERVUCAL CANCER:

Cervical cancer is a common types of slow-growing cancer in women that affects the mouth of the womb (uterus). The cervix connects the uterus to the vagina each year in the US, about 16,000 new cases of cervical cancer are diagnosed. The condition may start with changes in the shape, size or formation of cervical cells called Dysphasia.

SYMPTOMS:

Pre-cancerous cervical conditions are generally painless. They are not easily detected unless the patient has a pelvic exam and a Pap smear. Symptoms include:

- Abnormal bleeding. This happens only after the cervical cells become cancerous and invade neighboring tissues.

- Unusual vaginal discharge

- Increased bleeding during menstruation

- Bleeding between regular menstrual periods or after sexual intercourse, douching or a pelvic exam.

- Difficulty or pain in urination

- Pain during intercourse

- Pain in the pelvic area

- Pre-or post-menopausal bleeding.

These symptoms may also be caused by other less serious health problems. Patients are encouraged to visit their doctors when experiencing similar symptoms.

CAUSES AND RISK FACTORS:

A virus called human papillomavirus (HPV) is believed to cause cells and tissues in the cervix to grow abnormally to develop into cervical cancer. About 6 million women in the U. S. are infected with HPV. While researchers work to learn more about this form of cancer, certain risk factors are known:

- Having many sexual partners

- First intercourse at a young age

- History of smoking DIAGNOSIS:

Pelvic exams, Pap smears and biopsies are methods used to detect cervical and abnormal, pre-cancerous cervix lesions.

A pelvic exam involves the doctor probing for lumps abnormalities in shape of size of the uterus vagina, ovaries, fallopian tubes, bladder and rectum using a speculum. This instrument enlarges the vagina and allows the doctor to see the upper portion of the vagina and the cervix.

A pap smear is a simple and painless test often done during a pelvic exam. A small wooden scraper (spatula) and/or a small brush is used to collect cell samples from, the upper portion of the vagina and the cervix. Samples are looked at under a microscope to check for abnormal cells. Pap smears examine only cervical cells and are not indicators of uterine cancer.

Biopsy requires a doctor scraping or removing a small amount of tissue from the cervix while the patient is under anesthesia. The sample is sent to the laboratory to see if cancer cells are present.

TREATMENT

After test and examination results are in, the doctor will discuss with the patient what treatments will likely work best for her condition. Treatment plans depend on the following:

- Patient's age

- Patient's general health

- Tumor size

- Stage of the disease

- Speed of cell growth and degree of spreading (tumor grade)

- Effect of female hormones on tumor size

- Patient's desire to have children in the future

TREATMENTFOR CERVICAL CANCER INCLUDE:

- Surgery

- Radiation therapy

- Chemotherapy

- Biologic Therapy

WHAT EXACTLY IS HUMAN PAPILLOMA VIRUS?

According to the gentle soft Spanish-speaking oncologist, Dr. M. P. Medina of Kaiser Permanente, HPV is a common virus. He stated that as reported by the Center for Disease Control, 29 million people in the United States had the virus in 2005.

There are many different types of HPV, some causes no harm. Others can cause disease of the genital area. For most people, the virus goes away on its own. When the virus does not go away, it can develop into cervical cancer, pre-cancerous lesions, or genital warts depending on the HPV type.

Cancer of the cervix is a serious disease that can be life threatening. This disease is caused by certain HPV types that can cause the cells in the lining of the cervix to change form normal to pre-cancerous lesions. If these are not treated, they can turn cancerous. Gardisil is given in three doses injections.

* First at a date chosen by you and your health care provider. Second dose is two months after the first dose. - Third dose is given six months after the first dose.

Dr. Medina reminded us that getting the vaccine, does not mean that close and regular check-ups with your doctor is r still strongly advised.

Before we learn more about the various types of cancer its causes symptoms treatments and outcome, I would like for you to learn about particular disease, and how you can help your doctor make your journey through this valley of fear more optimistic.

COLORECTAL CANCER:

Colorectal cancer affects the digestive system. This includes the large and small intestines.

The large intestine is also called the colon.

Colorectal cancer is the third leading cause of cancer related deaths in the United States among both men and women. For men, only lung and prostate cancers show higher numbers. In women, only lung and breast cancers outrank colorectal cancer.

The intestines break down and absorbs food and water. They also carry away the body's digestive waste products. Genetic screening can help determine if patients may be at risk for getting the disease.

COLORECTAL CANCER SYMPTOMS

Adenocarcinoma of the colon and rectum grows slowly. A long time may pass before it becomes large enough to cause symptoms. Routine exams are important for early diagnosis.

When symptoms do occur, they vary depending on the location of the tumor, its type, how far it has spread and complications it may have caused.

On the right-hand side of the colon, blockage usually doesn't occur until later stages. This is because the space inside the colon is large, the colon wall is fairly thin and the material passing through is mostly liquid. Some tumors may grow big enough to be felt from the outside of the body. If there is bleeding inside it usually isn't obvious However, a person may feel weak or tired because of severe anemia caused by loss of blood.

On the left-hand side of the colon, the space inside the colon is smaller and the material that passes through it is semi-solid. Colon cancer can cause both constipation and diarrhea. A person may feel cramp-like pain in the stomach. The stool may be streaked or mixed with blood.

In rectal cancer, the most common symptom is usually bleeding when going to the bathroom. Cancer of the rectum should be considered whenever there is rectal bleeding, even if other causes such as hemorrhoids are present. A person may feel as if there is incomplete evacuation. There usually is no pain until later stages of the condition.

SYMPTOMS OF ADVANCED DISEASE INCLUDE:

- A feeling of being full very quickly while eating

- Weakness and pain in the abdominal area

- CAUSES AND RISK FACTORS

- There is no single cause of intestinal cancer. Several risk factors may play a role in its development.

- Person's betweens the ages of 40 and 75 are at greater risk of getting colorectal cancer than younger people. More women get colon cancer. More men get rectal cancer.

- Conditions such as familial polypasis, Lymph syndrome, Cohn's disease or Ulcerative colitis (ulcers in the lining of the large intestines) tend to increase the risk for the disease. Brothers, sisters and children of those already diagnosed with colorectal cancer have a greater chance of getting the disease later in life.

Population groups who have a high rate of colorectal cancer tend to eat low-fiber diets high in animal protein, fat and refined carbohydrates. The exact way the condition occurs is not yet known.

DIAGNOSIS

Screening is very effective for detecting early stages of colorectal cancer. Starting at age 40, even people who have no risk factors and no symptoms should have a digital rectal exam and a test for blood in the stool every year. At age 50, everyone should have a sigmoidoscopy or a similar test. Screening tests include:

- Digital rectal exam. The doctor inserts a gloved finger into the rectum to feel for lumps and to check for blood in the stool.

- Sigmoidoscopy. An instrument called a sigmoidoscope is inserted to look inside the rectum and part of the colon.

- Colonoscopy. An instrument called colon scope is used to examine the rectum and the entire colon.

- Computed tomography scan. A special X-ray create:? a computerized picture of the colon and rectum.

- Barium enema. A liquid is inserted into the rectum, and a series of X-rays are taken. This allows doctors to look for abnormal growths in the colon and rectum.

- Biopsy. If these results are abnormal, the doctor may examine a small piece of the tumor under the microscope.

- Genetic risk assessment. This is a method of identifying genes that may increase this chance of getting certain diseases.

TREATMENT:

The main treatment for colon cancer is surgery. The; part of the large bowel with cancer is removed, along with surrounding lymph nodes. The remaining bowel is joined together. Surgery is a cure for 70% of patients with colon cancer. Persons who have cancer that is limited to the mucous lining of the colon have the best chance of survival. Persons who have cancer in the lymph nodes have a less optimistic outlook.

Treatment of rectal cancer depends on how far the tumor has spread and how close it is to the rectum.

If there is not enough healthy colon to reconnect after the tumor is removed, the person may need a colostomy. This is rarely permanent. For this procedure is surgical opening is made in the abdomen and the end of the bowel is placed through the hole. A bag is placed over the opening to collect the stool.

A combination of radiation therapy and chemotherapy may be helpful for rectal cancer patients, especially if one to four lymph nodes are affected. Careful planning and attention is given to avoid injury to the small intestine.

Follow-up care with the surgeon, gastroenterologist and oncologist is important. The most common time of cancer recurs is within the first two years following diagnosis and treatment.

Periodic checkups may include a physical exam, blood tests, and colonoscopy, CT scan or PET scan.

The frequency of follow-up after surgery varies. Most experts recommend two annual inspections of the remaining bowel with colonoscopy or X-rays. If results are negative, repeat evaluations may be done at two to three-year intervals.

When it is not possible to remove the cancer entirely, surgery may be helpful in managing symptoms. Chemotherapy can be used for advanced colon cancer to slow progression of the disease

BELOW IS AN ILLUSTRATION OF THE ACTUAL COLON TUMOR FOUND IN MY ASCENDING COLON IN MARCH 2006. THE INITIAL COLONOSPOPY AND BIOPSY DETERMINED THAT THE TUMOR WAS BENIGN, BUT THE SIZE WAS PHENOMINAL. A

STOOL SPECIMEN ALSO PROVED NEGATIVE FOR BLOOD IN THE STOOL, THAT TOO WAS NEGATIVE.. BUT MY RED BLOOD COUNT WAS EXTREMELY LOW, AND SEVERAL IRON INFUSIONS WERE ADMINISTERED.

IN NOVEMBER OF 2006, IT WAS DECIDED THAT THE TUMOR SHOUOD BE REMOVED WITH ELECTRONIC INSTRUMENTS, SINCE I HAVE COPD, AND CONGESTIVCE HEART DISEASE, AND GENERAL ANESTHESIA SHOULD NOT BE ADMINISTERED.

The surgeon's attempt failed, but as you can see, he was able to cut away many parts of the large tumor, for testing and disposal. The fo11owing biopsy also was benign. With determination, the surgical team decided that if this tumor remained in my colon, at the rate it was growing, it would eventually block the entire colon.

A LAPOROTOMY WAS SCHEDULED UNDER GENERAL ANESTHESIA, WITH A VERY PLEASANT, AND CONCERNED DOCTOR NAMED Rupp. A lot of emergency equipment was gathered in the operating room, as well as lung, and heart specialist on call. That hugh mass was removed successfully, and I made a miraculous recovery.

SEVEN DAYS AFTER SURGERY, MY SURGEON,. AND INTERNAL MEDI CINE DOCTORS APPROVED MY ANNUAL FAMILY REUNION IN LAS VEGAS.

MY HUSBAND, AND TWO OF MY GROWN CHILDREN DROVE, AND WE HAD A SPLENDID TIME.

WE STAYED AT THE ORLEANS HOTEL WHICH IS NOT ON THE STRIP, AND IT HAS A COMPLETE ENTERTAINMENT CENTER INSIDE THE STRUCTURE, WHICH INCLUIDED BOWLING, A MOVIE THEATRE, SHOPPING STORES, AN INTERNATIONAL BUFFET WHERE WE MET EACH DY FOR BREAKFAST AT EIGHT AM, LUNCH AT TWELVE THIRTY, AND DINNER AT SIX PM. THE FOOD COURT WAS AN INTERNATIONAL SECTION OF AMERICAN BOOTHS REGULAR AND SOUTHERN, MEXICAN, ASIAN, FRENCH, GERMAN, AND OTHER COUNTRY'S TEMPTING OFFERINGS.

THERE WERE SEVERAL CLUBS FOR ENTERTAINMENT, BUT MY FAMILY MADE ME GO TO BED AND RELAX.

WHEN I RETURNED FOR MY PHYSICAL CHECK-UP, Dr. Rupp TOLD US THAT THERE WAS CANCER ON THE BACK SIDE OF THE TUMOR, CLASS II, BUT IT HAD NOT INVADED THE LYMPH NODES OR LIVER.

SEE TUMOR BELOW

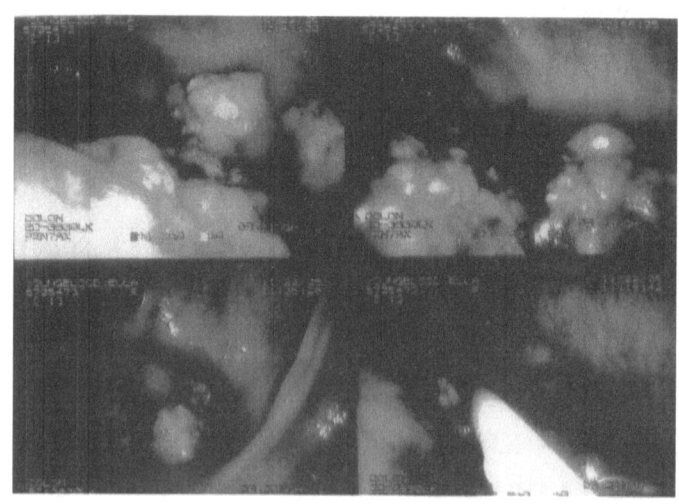

ESOPHAGEAL CANCER

The esophagus links the mouth to the stomach, forming an important part of the body's digestive system. Esophageal cancer includes lymphoma and tumors of the smooth muscles of the esophagus (which are usually not cancerous). The disease may show up as a narrowing of the esophagus, a lump or an abnormal flat area. Only about five percent of people with esophageal cancer survive more than five years.

SYMPTOMS

This disease is fairly rare. Its symptoms are usually subtle and inconsistent, including:

- Difficulty swallowing (solid foods first, then soft foods and eventually liquids)

- Pressure pain or burning in the chest

- Having swallowed food come back up (Regurgitation)

- Loosing a lot of weight. RISK FACTORS

African Americans are three times more likely than Caucasians to develop this type of cancer. Other risk factors include:

- Smoking and heavy alcohol use

- Cancer in another part of the body

- Swallowing lye or other chemicals

- Irritation from acid or bile backflow

- Conditions of the esophagus like Achalasia, Barrett 's esophagus or Plummer-vinson syndrome (esophageal web).

- Poor nutrition or a lack of trace minerals, particularly selenium

- Infections.

DIAGNOSIS

Cancer specialists have several techniques to help diagnose esophageal cancer;

- Barium swallow. The patient drinks a special liquid (barium), which travels trough the body and outlines the cancer when X-rayed.

- Biopsy. A special instrument (endoscopy) is used to take a sample of tissue, which is examined under a microscope.

- Endoscopic ultrasound, which allows the doctor to see if a mass has spread into the wall of the esophagus or nearby organs.

- Computed tomography (CT) scans to see if the tumor has spread to other organs, such as the liver or lungs.

TREATMENT

- Treatment usually involves a combination of options, specifically:

- Surgery

- Chemotherapy

- Radiation When the cancer is advanced, swallowing can be made easier by:

- Creating a passage through the tumor with expandable tubes tied can be opened up to allow food to pass through to the stomach.

- Laser therapy, which uses laser light to destroy abnormal tissues.

- Thermal coagulation therapy, which uses either a laser or a heater probe to destroy part of the tumor to let the patient swallow more easily.

KIDNEY CANCER

The kidneys are a pair of bean-shaped organs located on either side of the spine at about the waistline. These organs filter the blood and get rid of excess water, salt and waste products. Each kidney has a tube that carries urine to the bladder, where it is stored temporarily. Kidneys may develop cysts that are hollow, no cancerous growths or tumors that are cancerous.

There are three main types of kidney cancer:

- Renal cell, or cancer of the tube linings. This type accounts for about 80 percent of all kidney cancers.

- Wilm's tumor. This occurs mainly in children under five years old.

- Transitional cell cancer. This type develops in the linings of other digestive system areas.

SYMPTOMS

Signs of kidney cancer include:

- Blood in the urine, visible or microscopic

- Pain in the side of the body, accompanied by fever

- High blood pressure. Kidney cancer is often discovered during an examination related to this or other conditions.

CAUSES AND RISK FACTORS

- Most kidney cancers occur between the ages of 50 and 70

- Men are 1.5 times as likely to get the disease as women

- Smoking doubles the risk of developing the renal cell form of the Cancer.

- Exposure to asbestos, cadmium and certain chemicals

- Family history of kidney cancer

- Long-term kidney dialysis

- Being overweight, and eating a high-fat diet.

DIAGNOSIS

The following methods are used to diagnose kidney cancer

- Physical examination

- Ultrasound

- Whole body computed tomography (CT) scan. Or computed tomography scan of the abdomen.

- Magnetic resonance imaging (MRI) scan

- Special X-rays may be done before surgery to check the tumor and the arteries that supply it.

- TREATMENT

If the cancer has not spread to other parts of the body, removing it along with surrounding lymph nodes offers a good chance of cure. Most commonly, however kidney cancer spreads early, especially to the lungs. When this happens, neither Surgery, radiation nor chemotherapy can offer a cure.

LEUKEMIA

An estimated 27,000 new cases of leukemia are diagnosed annually. Leukemia is a cancer of the blood and bone marrow. Bone marrow is the sponge-like material found inside the large bones in the body. Bone marrow makes white blood cells (to prevent infection), platelets (to make the blood clot) and red blood cells (to carry oxygen and other materials to various parts of the body). Immature cells produced by the bone marrow are called blasts. Leukemia, blasts may fail to develop into mature cells, or they may not mature correctly.

Depending on the type of cells affected by the disease, the patient may develop one of four major types of lleukemia: **acute myelogenous leukemia** (AML), **acute lymphocyte leukemia (ALL), chronic myelogenous leukemia (CML) or chronic lymphocyte leukemia (CLL).** Leukemia can be generally divided into two groups, acute and chronic.

ACUTE LEUKEMIA

In acute leukemia, the disease spreads quickly as many undeveloped malignant blasts replace normal cells in the blood and marrow. The cancerous cells eventually stop producing red blood cells, white blood cells and/or platelets. The patient becomes anemic and gets infections. Having too few platelets prevents injuries from healing and makes the patient bleed easily.

CHRONIC LEUKEMIA

In chronic leukemia, the disease grows slowly and many more mature-looking cancer cells are found. A patient with chronic leukemia does not experience the same symptoms as the patient with acute leukemia, and treatment for the two kinds of leukemia is different.

SYMPTOMS

In its early stages the disease may not cause any symptoms at all. However, the following are possible signs of leukemia:

- Flu or cold symptoms

- Tiredness and shortness of breath when exerting physical effort

- Pale complexion from anemia

- Signs of bleeding caused by a very low platelet count, including black and blue marks occurring for no reason because of a minor injury; pinhead-sized spots appearing under the skin (petechlea): or prolonged bleeding from minor cuts.

- Mild fever, swollen gums, frequent minor infections like (pustules or sores in the anal area

- Slow healing of cuts

- Discomfort in bones or joints

- Enlarged liver and spleen

CAUSES AND RISK FACTORS

The causes of most forms of leukemia are not known,. Researchers believe the disease is due to complex interactions between genetic factors and the environment. Certain viruses are also suspected as promoting leukemia. The disease is not considered contagious or inherited. Risk factors include:

- Certain types of work may cause leukemia due to constant exposure to hazardous materials. Included are farmers involved in high levels of soybean production, cattle ranching dairy production and herbicide use; rubber manufacturing worker; asbestos workers and tire repair workers.

- Certain drugs used to treat other forms of cancers like breast cancer, ovarian cancer or lymphoma.

- Exposure to certain chemicals, such as benzene and some types of pesticides.

- Exposure to high doses of high-energy -rays (radiation).

DIAGNOSIS

The doctor may order blood counts for signs of leukemia. If red blood cell and platelet counts are low and suspicious blast cells can be seen, the doctor may perform a bone marrow biopsy. While the patient is under anesthesia, a large needle is inserted into the bone to remove a small amount of bone marrow. This is examined for the presence of abnormal blast cells, and the biopsy may find defects in genetic materials (chromosomes) linked to certain types of leukemia (for example, Philadelphia chromosome in CNL). The doctor will then be able to determine the type of leukemia present and design a plan for the most effective treatment.

TREATMENT

The approach to treating leukemia is different for each major type of leukemia.

- Biologic therapy

- Blood and marrow transplantation

- Chemotherapy

- Radiation therapy

LYMPHOMA

Lymphoma is one of the most common causes of death from cancer in the United States, and about 48,000 new cases of lymphoma are diagnosed every year. In lymphoma, cancer cells are found in the lymphatic system, which is comprised of the bone marrow, lymph nodes, spleen, stomach, intestines and skin. Because lymph tissues are present in many parts of the body, lymphoma can start almost anywhere.

LYMPH NODES

Normal lymph nodes are tiny, bean-like structures that trap cells containing poisons and waste materials. They also serve as a reservoir of cells that supply microorganism fighting antibodies Tube-like vessels carrying milk-colored fluid called lymph connect lymph nodes to each other. Lymph allows white blood cells Parenthesisnodes) to circulate.

When white blood cells multiply abnormally, they cause masses to form and lymph nodes become enlarged. Some lymphomas may affect the bone marrow and interfere with its making of blood cells. The result is anemia, or low red blood cell count.

CLASSIFICATION OF LYMPHOMAS

Lymphomas are graded as low, intermediate and high depending on the kind of lymphoma cells present and how they affect lymph nodes and chromosomes. Some lymphomas grow faster and require specific treatment. Classifying them is complex because many kinds of lymphocyte cells can be involved.

LOW- GRADE LYMPHOMA

These grow so slowly that patients can live for many years mostly without symptoms, although some may experience pain from an enlarged lymph gland. After five to ten years, low-grade disorders begin to progress rapidly to become aggressive or high-grade and produce more severe symptoms.

INTERMEDIATE-GRADE LYMPHOMA

This type progresses fairly rapidly, without treatment: With treatment, remission can be induced in between 50% to 75% of cases. Initial treatment has been so successful that people who stay in remission for three years after diagnosis are often considered cured. Stage 1 disorders are treated with radiotherapy.

HIGH-GRADE LYMPHOMA

Without treatment, these can progress rapidly regardless of stage. They are treated aggressively with treatment; between 50% to 75% of patients enter remission. Those who stay in remission one year can look forward to a life free from recurrence. Treatment consist of intensive combination chemotherapy, which is sometimes supplemented with radiation therapy. Drug regiments used are determined by a number of factors the most imposing being tissue study.

TYPES OF LYMPHOMAS

Based on the course of disease and the kind of lymphocytes affected, lymphomas are divided into two types: HODGKIN'S DISEASE and NON-HODGKIN'S LYMPJOPMA

HODGKIN'S DISEASE:

About 75% of those diagnosed with Hodgkin's disease recover fully. About 90% of all people diagnosed with early-stage illness and more than 50% of those with more advance stage are now living longer than 10 years with no signs of the disease coming back.

The stage of the disease at diagnosis is critical in planning treatments. Sometimes giving the patient aggressive chemotherapy and then introducing young cells from the bone marrow (bone marrow transplantation) may increase chances of one patient living longer. A bone marrow transplant should be considered for every patient whose disease comes back after undergoing chemotherapy.

NON-HODGKIN'S LYMPHOMA

In the last 10 years, this disease has become easier to treat, as more procedures are found to be effective. Overall, 59% to 60% of patients with NHL now live five years or longer without a recurrence. While a number of factors determine the best treatment for these disorders, the most significant is tissue classification followed by determination of the disease's stage.

SYMPTOMS

In most cases, patients consult their doctors if they have painless swelling in the neck, armpits, groins, or abdomen. Sometimes the swelling or the tumor occur in other organs, such as the skin or stomach (extra nodal lymphoma) either as a first symptom or a sign appearing later in the disease. Like most cancers, lymphoma is best treated when found early. Symptoms are:

- Loss of appetite

- Loss of weight, nausea, vomiting, indigestion or pain in the abdomen.

- A feeling of bloating

- Itching, bone pain, headaches constant coughing and abnormal pressure and congestion in the face, neck and upper chest.

- Fatigue and flu-like body aches

- Fatigue resulting from anemia

- Night sweats, recurring high-grade fever or constant low-grade fever.

CAUSES AND RISK FACTORS

The cause of lymphoma is still not known, but it is not considered hereditary. Most lymphomas occur between the ages of 40 and 70 years. Hodgkin's disease, considered the most curable form of lymphoma, often occurs in young adults or the elderly. Possible triggers for lymphoma include:

- Genetic factors

- Certain infections or environmental factors

- Exposure to herbicides and high doses of radiation (including aggressive radiation therapy)

- Certain viruses (human retroviruses like HTLV-1 and to some extent, the Epstein-Bar virus are also suspected)

- AIDS (acquired immunodeficiency syndrome). These patients require specialized treatment.

- Abnormalities in the genetic materials called chromosomes and the body's immune response.

- Although the disease has been reported in patients who live or work physically close to each other (clustering), no evidence exists that indicate the disease is infectious

DIAGNOSIS

In reaching a diagnosis of lymphoma, doctors may do the following:

- Take the patient's medical history

- Conduct a thorough physical examination to detect an enlarged lymph node, liver and/or spleen

- Order blood tests to check kidney and liver functioning

- Do a biopsy by removing a small amount of tissue from the suspected area and examining it to see the type of lymphoma present.

TREATMENT

Radiotherapy is the preferred treatment for patients with stage I or II lymphomas because it successfully induces long-term remissions and *even* cures in many diseases. For treatment of stage III or IV low-grade disorders, one school of thought is to start intensive therapy right after diagnosis. - When a patient has lymphomas or not - to achieve and maintain complete remission. Treatment usually consists of high-dose radiotherapy, chemotherapy or a combination of both. Intensive treatment involves risk, but recent studies suggest that such a treatment may induce; high rates of remission.

Bone marrow transplant is currently being studied as a treatment option for low-grade lymphoma.

MESOTHELIOMA

Malignant mesothelioma is a rare cancer that affects tee cells lining various organs of the body, particularly in the chest, abdomen and the heart. These cells grow rapidly and can eventually encase the involved organ.

SYMPTOMS

Malignant mesothelioma may not become apparent until 20 to 30 years after the first exposure to asbestos. Symptoms include:

- Difficulty breathing, pain in the chest or both

- Hoarseness, difficulty swallowing or coughing up of blood

- Increase in waist size or abdominal pain if cancer cells are growing,,

CAUSES AND RISK FACTORS

Mesothelioma is most commonly diagnosed in patients 50 to60 years of age. It occurs five times more often in men than women, Risk factors include:

- Exposure to asbestos. Needle-shaped asbestos fibers that cannot be cleared by the lungs cause cells to become cancerous.

- Exposure to beryllium and zeolite. (Any of various natural or synthesized silicates of similar structure used in water softening and as adsorbents).

DIAGNOSIS

Mesothelioma can be diagnosed through several tests, including:

- X-rays. Chest or abdominal X-rays can detect an accumulation of fluid in the lungs or abdomen.

- Fluid sample examination. Doctors look for a substance called carcinoernbronic antigen (CEA)- high levels of which may suggest the presence of lung cancer rather than mesothelioma.

- Biopsy. To confirm the diagnosis a sample of tissue may be taken for examination under the microscope.

- Computed tomography (CT) scans. These scans check other parts of the body for the disease through use of a computerized image.

TREATMENT

Because of the aggressive nature of malignant mesothelioma, treatment is difficult. Therapy may include a combination of surgery, radiation therapy, chemotherapy and photodynamic therapy. The amount of tissue removed during surgery is determined by the extent of the tumor.

- Radiation therapy. This treatment involves the administration of X-ray to the affected tissues for a specified period of time.

- Chemotherapy. Drugs, such as caboplatin, cisplatin or doxorubicin, are injected into the veins every three to four weeks.

- Photodynamic therapy. Administering photoferin II causes the cells to die when it is activated with a special light.

MYELODYSPLASTIC SYNDROMES (MDS)

- Myelodysplastic syndromes affect blood cell production and behavior. Blood carries oxygen chemicals and hormones to the cells in the body and helps remove toxins and waste. Bone marrow (the spongy middle; part of the large bones) produces the three main types of blood cells:

- Red blood cells carry oxygen to the tissues (muscles, bones, nerves and organs). Low red blood counts or malfunctioning red blood cells can cause anemia Symptoms are paleness, feeling tired, fast-beating or pounding heart, dizziness, shortness of breath, or headaches.

- White blood cells fight infection. Symptoms of infection caused by low white blood counts may include temperature rising to 38.0 C or 100.4 F, coughing, stiff neck, pain or burning with urination, sore throat, mouth or lip sores and sores that do not heal.

- Platelets help to prevent bleeding. Signs of inadequate plates include bleeding or bruising too easily. Patients may experience bleeding of the gums when brushing or visual changes or a stiff neck. *THE FIVE CATEGORIES OF MDS ARE:*

    - *Refractory anemia*

    - *Refractory anemia with ringed sideroblasts*

- *Refractory anemia with excess blasts*

- *Refractory anemia in transformation to acute leukemia*

- *Chronic myelomonocytic leukemia*

The disease categories on the lower end of this list are more serious and have a worse prognosis than those at the top. Refractory anemia and refractory anemia with ringed side oblasts primarily affect the red blood cells and are the most common forms of MDS. Refractory anemia with excess blasts is present when immature white blood cells are found in the bone marrow in abnormally large numbers (five to 20% bone marrow blasts, compared to normal blasts of less than one percent). Refractory anemia with excess blasts in transformation occurs when blasts become markedly increased (more than 20%) and may indicate that MDS will change to an acute form of leukemia.

SYMPTOMS

When symptoms appear they are usually subtle. MDS may remain stable for several years, or it may get worse quickly and progress to acute myeloid leukemia. The most common symptoms are:

- Signs of anemia, such as weakness, tiredness, headaches, heart palpitations and dizziness.

- Low platelet counts cause easy and profuse bleeding, as well as unexplained bruising.

- Women may experience heavy menstrual periods.

- Susceptibility to infection due to low number of white blood cells.

CAUSES AND RISK FACTORS

- MDS may begin without any apparent cause possible risk factors include:

    - Exposure to certain chemicals, such as pesticides

    - Exposure to chemotherapy, or non-chemotherapy drugs and radiation

    - Age may also be a factor since MDS is most commonly diagnosed in people 60 and older.

MDS IS DIFFICULT TO DIAGNOSE   BECAUSE OF THE ABSENCE OF SYMPTOMS IN THE EARLY STAGE OF THE DISEASE. Often it is accidentally discovered during a routine physical exam or blood test. Routine screening tests do not exist for MDS, but if the disease is suspected, the doctor may order these tests:

- Complete blood count. A small amount of blood is drawn from the arm, and the lab measures red blood cells, white blood cells and platelets in the sample.

- Bone marrow biopsy

- An examination of the chromosomes that carry genetic material

TREATMENT

MDS is a progressive disease as bone marrow becomes more affected, blood cells become more abnormal. Since no current therapies are effective in preventing MDS from worsening, treatment usually focuses on relieving the symptoms. Doctors will discuss with the patient the various options available, including:

- Antibiotics

- Red blood cell or platelet transfusions

- Chemotherapy

- Biologic therapy

- Differentiating agents (DRUGS)

- Bone marrow transplant

- Leukemia treatment MDS may change into acute myelogenous leukemia (AML), AML causes large numbers of immature white blood cells to be produced by the bone marrow. When this occurs, the patient is treated for AML rather than MDS, Patients with refractory anemia with excess blasts and chronic myelomonocytic leukemia have a higher risk of progression.

OVARIAN CANCER

In the female body, two ovaries (each about an inch-and -half long) are located on the left and right sides of the uterus in the pelvic region. Ovaries produce hormones and hold egg cells, which can develop into a fetus when fertilized.

Each year more than 22,000 women in the United States learn that they have ovarian cancer.

When cancer cells are found in the lining of the ovary the condition is called epithelial ovarian cancer. When malignant cells and tumor are found in the egg producing cells , the condition is called germ cell ovarian cancer. Genetic screening can help determine if a woman is a carrier of a mutated (changed) gene and, therefore , at greater risk of developing the disease.

SYMPTOMS

Often no symptoms are evident in the early stages of the disease. When symptoms appear, they may include;

- Gas, nausea, indigestion that does not go away

- Frequent urination

- Unexplained change in bowel habits

- Abnormal postmenopausal bleeding

- Weight gain or loss

- Pain during intercourse

- Abdominal swelling and/or pain, bloating or a feeling of fullness. Ovarian cancer may spread to the sac inside the abdomen that holds the intestines, uterus and ovaries, causing fluid to accumulate and the abdomen to swell.

- Shortness of breath caused by the spread of the disease to the muscle under the lung. Fluid buildup in the area makes it difficult for the patient to breathe.

If symptoms continue for longer than four to six weeks, patients should insist on a thorough pelvic examination by their doctor.

RISK FACTORS

- A family history of the disease, especially in a mother, daughter or sister

- Family history of breast or colon cancer

- Being a woman older than age 50

- Never having had children

- Having taken certain fertility drugs

DIAGNOSIS

A comprehensive medical history is taken, and a physical exam (including a pelvic examination) is performed. For this, the doctor inserts one gloved finger in the rectum and one in the vagina at the same time. The vagina, rectum and lower abdomen are probed for masses and growths. Taking a mild laxative or enema before the pelvic exam can be helpful. Other tests include:

- A Pap smear (a common test for career of the cervix) is often part of the pelvis exam, though it does not offer a reliable way to diagnose ovarian cancer. Every woman should undergo regular rectal and vaginal pelvic examinations.

- Transvaginal sonography and tumor markers are alternative ways of diagnosing ovarian cancer.

- Ultrosonography aims high frequency sound waves at the ovaries. The echo pattern produced creates a picture called a sonogram. Healthy tissues, fluid-filled cysts and tumors produce different echoes.

- A computed topography (CT or CAT) scan, a series of computerized X-rays, allows doctors to see cancer cells.

- A lower GI series, or barium enema, is a series of X-rays of the colon and rectum. Pictures are taken after the patient is given an enema with a white chalky solution containing barium. The barium outlines the colon and the rectum on the X-ray, which helps the doctor see tumors or other abnormal areas.

- An intravenous pyelogram (IVP) is an X-ray of the kidneys and uterus taken when dye is injected into the body.

- Blood tests measure a substance in the blood called CA-125. Ovarian cancer cells can produce this tumor marker. CA-125 is not always present in women with ovarian cancer, though it may be present in women who have benign ovarian conditions. This blood test cannot be used alone to diagnose cancer.

A biopsy (removing and examining tissue) of the ovaries is the only way to definitively diagnose cancer. If cancer is suspected, the surgeon removes the entire ovary (oophorectomy) because infected cells could escape and spread when cutting through the outer layer of the ovary. The surgeon also removes nearby lymph noses, samples of tissue from the diaphragm and other organs and fluid from the abdomen. A pathologist examines these cells to identify cancer. This process, called surgical staging, is needed to find out whether the cancer has spread and to determine a plan for treatment.

TREATMENT

Treating ovarian cancer depends on a number of factor, including the stage of the disease and the woman's age and general health. Oncologists who specialize in this disease can best determine the treatment plan. Because treatment decisions are complex, more than one doctor's advice can be helpful.

When talking about choices, the patient may want to ask about taking part in a research study or clinical trial. These scientific studies are designed to find new and better ways to treat cancer. Ovarian cancer treatment possibilities are:

- Surgery to remove the uterus, both ovaries and the fallopian tubes.

- Chemotherapy (anti-cancer drugs)

- Radiation therapy (Also called radiotherapy.

PANCREATIC CANCER

Nearly 30,000 people are diagnosed with pancreatic cancer in the United States every year and most die from the disease. Pancreatic cancer is the fifth-leading cause of adult cancer-related deaths in the United States. This cancer usually occurs in people over the age of 65 and is rarely seen in persons under 45. The pancreas is a gland located in the abdomen that produces several hormones, including insulin. Pancreatic secretions aid the digestion of food and help the *body* to use glucose, (sugar).

It strikes men and women equally. Like so many other cancers, the earlier it's caught, the greater the chances of survival. However, there is no screening test available for pancreatic cancer. By the time symptoms appear it's usually too late for a cure.

SYMPTOMS

The symptoms of pancreatic cancer are often vague or not apparent making the disease difficult to diagnose. Frequently, it reaches an advanced stage before symptoms occur. The most common are:

- Abdominal pain

- Loss of appetite, nausea or weight loss

- Jaundice (a yellowish discoloration of the skin and whites of the eyes)

- Back pain

- Feeling of weakness

CAUSES AND RISK FACTORS

An individual's risk of getting pancreatic cancer increase if he or she;

- Uses tobacco

- Eats a high fat diet

- Has chronic pancreatitis

- Has a hereditary form of pancreatitis or pancreatic cancer

- Works with metals or chemicals

- Is African American

DIAGNOSIS

The exocrine part of the pancreas (which produces the digestive fluids that help break down fats, proteins and carbohydrates) is where 95% of all pancreatic cancers, or adenocarcinomas, begin. The other five percent grow in the endocrine section, where hormones (like insulin) are made identifying the type of tumor is important since they may, develop and respond to treatment differently, Pancreatic cancer's symptoms are like those of many other pancreatic conditions. That's why it's important to be seen by an expert who may use any of the following tests for an accurate diagnosis:

- Basic blood test and a lab test called CA19-9.

- Ultrasound. Though not a definitive test for tumors it is a good way to find gallstones or cysts in the pancreas.

- Computed topography (CT) scans. These three-dimensional X-rays are accurate tests for cancer. A CT scan is also used to guide a biopsy needle exactly to the tumor to take a tissue sample for lab analysis.

- Magnetic resonance imaging (MRI) This uses magnetic fields and radio waves to create detailed images of soft tissue. A special type, magnetic resonance cholagioancreatography (MRCP), can find blockages in the pancreatic and bile ducts.

* Endoscopic retrograde cholanfiopancreatography (ERCP). This minimally invasive procedure is considered the gold standard for pancreatic and billary diagnosis, but there is a two to five percent risk of causing pancreatitis.

Currently, there are no affective screening tests to detect pancreatis comer it is often difficult for a doctor to distinguish between pancreatitis (inflammation of the pancreas) and pancreatic cancer. Both conditions present similar symptoms and may look the same

On radiology scans. Most patients require exploratory surgery to establish a diagnosis of pancreatic cancer and determine the extent of the disease,

TREATMENT

Treatment for pancreatic cancer includes surgery, chemotherapy, radiation therapy or a combination, depending on the stage of the disease.

Exploratory surgery is performed through an incision in the abdomen (laperotomy). This allows the surgeon to assess the extent of the disease. If the tumor can be removed, a Whipple procedure (pancreatoduodenectomy) is used, which can be very effective and results in few complications. Only five to 20% of patients have tumors that can be surgically removed. Laparoscopy, a less invasive procedure, is sometimes done. The surgeon inserts a laparoscope (flexible telescope with a camera attached) into the abdomen to see how far the disease has progressed.

Chemotherapy or radiation may benefit the patient if the tumor cannot be removed. Neither can be done until the patient has sufficiently recovered from the exploratory surgery, which usually takes about six weeks.

SKIN CANCER

Skin cancer is the most common of all cancers. Between 40 to 50% of all cancers cases diagnosed every year are skin cancer. There are two main types of skin cancer: Malignant melanoma and nonmelanoma skin cancer

NONMELANOMA SKIN CANCER

The most common types are basal cell carcinoma and squamous cell carcinoma. Basal cell carcinoma forms in the thin, upper layer of the skin (epidermis). It is usually found on the sun-exposed areas of the body, such as the neck and head. About 75% of all skin cancers are of this type.

They are slow growing and do not usually spared. After treatment, basal cell carcinoma may grow again on the same spot or appear elsewhere on the skin. Between 35 to 50% of people who develop one basal cell carcinoma will grow a new skin cancer within five years of diagnosis.

Accounting for about 20% of all skin cancers squamous cell carcinomas also form on the top, thin layer of the skin and are commonly seen on sun-exposed areas such as the face neck, lips, neck or back of the hand. However, it can also develop in other locations, including the genital area. Squamous cell carcinoma is more aggressive than basal cell carcinoma and more likely to spread to other parts of the body.

Less common non melanomas (e.g.. Kaposi's sarcoma and cutaneous lymphoma) make up less than one percent of non melanoma cancers.

MELANOMA

Melanomas account for only four percent of all skin cancer cases but are far more dangerous. Of all skin cancer-related disease 79% are from melanoma. In this disease, cancer develops in cells (melanocytes) that produce skin pigmentation. A black or brown spot appears typically, on the torso of males and lower legs of females. It may also form on the palm of the hands soles of the feet and under the nails. Very rarely it appears in parts of the body not covered by skin, such as the mouth, eyes, vagina and internal organs. Melanoma is more likely than non melanoma skin cancer to spread to lymph nodes and other parts of the body.

SYMPTOMS

Non melanoma skin cancer may cause the following symptoms:

- Spots or bumps that grow over time (a few months to a year or two) or that appear as a sore that does not heal within three months.

- Basal cell carcinomas may appear as flat, firm, pale areas or small, raised, translucent, pink or red, shiny, waxy areas with visible blood vessels or depressed center areas that bleed when slightly injured.

- Large basal cell carcinomas have oozing, crusty areas.

- Squamous cell caracinomas may look like small lumps with uneven rough surface or flat reddish patch that slowly grows.

Melanoma skin cancer may appear as:

* Spots, sores, lumps. Blemishes or markings on the skin that change in shape, size or color.

Skin may become reddish, crusty or scaly.

Skin may ooze, bleed or swell or may feel painful, scratchy or tender.

CAUSES AND RISK FACTORS:

The following factors increase your risk of getting skin cancer:

Frequent exposure to ultraviolet (UV) rays. Sunlight is the main source of this exposure. Tanning lamps and tanning booths are other sources of UV radiation.

Fair skin, Caucasians are 20 times more likely to develop skin cancer than African Americans. Fair-skinned individuals with red or blonde hair and skin that freckles or burns easily are also at greater risk.

59 years or older. Half of all melanoma causes occur in this age group. However some melanoma cases also occur in people age 20 to 30 years. In fact the most common cancer among people under 30 years old is melanoma.

- Family history: Individuals whose immediate relatives (mother, father, sister, brother, child) have been diagnosed with melanoma are considered at high risk. About 10% of melanoma cases show a family history of the disease.

- Reduced immunity: Individuals who have received medications that suppress the immune system, such as organ transplant recipients, are more likely to develop melanoma.

- Male gender: Men are two times more likely than women to develop basal cell carcinoma and three times more likely to develop squamous cell carcinoma.

- Exposure of chemicals: Arsenic (an ingredient in pesticides), paraffin, industrial tar, coal and certain types of oil may increase risk.

- Exposure to radiation: Individuals who have undergone radiation treatment are at risk to develop nonmelanoma skin cancer in the irradiated area.

- Severe skin injury: Scarring from bums, bone infections and other severe inflammatory skin diseases are risk factors.

- Psoriasis treatment: Patients receiving psoralen and UV light treatment (PUVA) may be at risk.

Most people have moles, which are generally harmless. However, certain types can change in appearance, color or size and develop into melanoma. To distinguish between a normal mole and a melanoma, use the ABCD rule:

- Asymmetry: Half the mole looks different from the other half.

- Border: The edges of the mole are irregular or ragged.

- Color: Moles are non-uniform in color, and

- Diameter: Normal moles are typically smaller than six millimeters (a quarter inch) in diameter. Melanomas are generally bigger, although recently doctors have seen melanomas between three and six millimeters in diameter.

DIAGNOSIS

A Doctor will take a complete medical history and perform a physical exam. If abnormal markings are found, the doctor will perform additional tests. One such test is the biopsy, in which a skin sample is taken and examined in the lab. If lymph nodes are too large or too firm, a lymph node biopsy will also be done using a fine needle to remove a small piece of tissue from the suspected tumor. If this procedure does not indicate a clear result, a surgeon may remove the lymph node for further examination, usually in a doctor's office or at an outpatient clinic.

TREATMENT:

Skin cancer may be treated with surgery to remove the malignant area, chemotherapy, radiation therapy or a combination of all of these. The specific treatment will depend on the type of skin cancer how advanced it is, how aggressive it is, where it is located and the general health of the patient.

PREVENTION:

Skin cancer can be cured if detected early. The American Cancer Society recommends a cancer-related checkup with skin examination every three years for people 20 to 40 years old and annual exams for persons over 40.

Doctors suggest that patients perform monthly self-examinations in front of a full-length mirror. All areas of the body must be checked, including palms and soles, back of the torso and back of the legs. One out of three melanomas in men are on the back.

OTHER SIMPLE PRECAUTIONS ARE:

- Avoid being outdoors too long in intense sunlight. Peak hours to avoid are 10 a.m. to 3 p.m.

- Wear protective clothing when outdoors. You can protect yourself by simply wearing a shirt and a broad-rimmed hat.

- Use sunscreen. Sunscreen with SPF factor of 15 or higher, should be applied to sun exposed skin. Many sunscreens wear off from sweating or swimming and should be reapplied. Use sunscreen even on a hazy or cloudy day. Ultraviolet rays can still penetrate the atmosphere.

- Wear sunglasses: UV absorption of 99 to 100% is recommended to provide good protection for the eyes and the surrounding skin.

- Avoid other sources of UV light. Tanning beds and sun lamps can deliver damaging amounts of UV light to the skin and should be avoided or used lightly.

- Provide sun protection for children. Children should be cautioned about the harmful effects of excessive sun exposure. Parents should instill in their children the habit of using sunscreen and protective clothing *for* outdoor activities.

Learn more about skin cancer. Many organizations, including the National Institutes of Health and the American Cancer Society, provide public service and information materials.

STOMACH CANCER

Stomach cancer in the United States is the seventh most common cause of death from cancer. About 95 percent of all stomach cancer is gastric adenocarcinoma. Other, less common forms are lymphomas and leiomyosarcomas.

Adenoearcinoma is classified by how it looks:

- A pouch that juts out, like a polyp (A patient with this type of tumor has a better chance of survival than if the tumor is penetrating).

- A sharp, well-defined border that may be ulcerated

- Spreading, which spreads across the surface of the lining of the stomach or into its walls

- Miscellaneous, which means the tumor, shows characteristics of the other types (Most fall into this category.)

SYMPTOMS

In its early stage, stomach cancer has no specific symptoms. Both doctors and patients tend to dismiss any symptoms, often for months. Clues to the presence of stomach cancer include

- Feeling full after a large meal, which is more likely if the cancer is blocking the region where the stomach empties into the intestines

- Pain, which may suggest peptic ulcer

- Loss of weight or strength due to not getting enough nutrients.

Bleeding is rare, but it may cause anemia (low blood counts)., Occasionally the first symptoms of stomach cancer is evidence of its having spread to other organs. This may lead to an enlarged liver, jaundice, fluid accumulation in the spaces between tissues and organs in the abdominal cavity, skin nodules and bone fractures.

CAUSES AND RISK FACTORS

The cause of stomach cancer is not yet known. Gastric ulcers are sometimes thought to lead to cancer. H. pylori, a bacteria that causes ulcers, may be a factor leading to stomach cancer.

Gastritis and intestinal metaplasia of the gastric mucus are often found but are generally thought to be a result, rather than an early sign, of gastric cancer. Persons who have ulcers of the duodenum (the connection between the lower part of the stomach and the intestines) generally have a lower risk of getting stomach cancer.

DIAGNOSIS

One of she key elements of an accurate diagnosis is distinguishing stomach cancer from peptic ulcer and its complications. Some diagnostic procedures used include:

- Endoscopy, which allows the doctor to see the area aid take samples of tissue from suspicious areas.

- Examination of cells taken from the area or areas of concern.

- Double-contrast X-ray techniques in which the inside: of the stomach is coated with barium. The stomach is then inflated and examined using X-rays.

TREATMENT

The earlier the tumor is found, the more effective treatment is. The more superficial the tumor is when found, the better the results of treatment. Treatment of primary lymphomas is more effective than treatment of gastric Adeuacarcinoma.

Treatment, depending on the nature of the tumor, may include:

- Surgery, which involves removing most or all the stomach and adjacent lymph nodes. In some situations, when a patient's quality of life can be improved, surgery to bypass an obstructing tumor may be done.

- Combining chemotherapy and radiation therapy especially in gastric lymphoma

CHAPTER FOUR

I have received from the Massachusetts General Hospital Cancer Center in Boston, the alphabetical methods of helping you find your cancer type

Find Your Cancer Type by Body System ABCDEFGHIJKLMNOPQ RSTUVWXZ

Cancer can be grouped by body system. For example, colon cancer is considered a Gastrointestinal cancer, and Kidney cancer is Genitourinary

DIAGNOSIS	CANCER TYPE
Acute Lymphoblastic Leukemia (ALL)	**Leukemia**
Acute Myeloid Leukemia (AML)	**Leukemia**
Adrenal Cancer of	Adrenal Cancer
Aids-related Lymphoma	Aids Related Cancers
Aids-related malignancies	Aids-related cancers
Alveolar Soft Part Sarcoma	Soft Tissue Sarcoma
Anal Cancer	Anal Cancer
Anaplastic Astrocyloma	Brain Tumors
Anaplastic Carcinoma Thyroid	Thyroid
Angiosarcoma	Soft Tissue Sarcoma
Astrocytomas/Glioma	Brain Tumors
Atypical Teraloid Rhabdoid Tumor	Brain Tumors

B

Basal Cell Carcinoma	Basal Cell, and Squamous Cell Carcinoma

Liver Cancer
Bladder Cancer
Metastatic Cancer
Brain Tumors
Brain Tumors
Breast Cancer
Male Breast Cancer
Lrymphoma
Bile Duct Cancer
Bladder Cancer
Bone Cancer Metastatic Brain Cancer

Brain Stem Glioma Breast Cancer
Burkitt's Lymphoma

C
Cancer of Unknown Primary (cup)
Cancer of Unkniown Primary
Carcinoid Tumor   Carcoid Tumor
Cervical Cancer   Cervical Cancer
Cholangiocarcinoma (Cancer of the
Bile Duct) Liver Cancer
Chondromsarcoma   Soft Tissue Sarcoma
Chordoma   Brain Tumors
Choroid Plexus Tumors   Brain Tumors
Chronic Lymphocite Leulemia (CLL)
Leukemia
Chronic Mylogenous Leukemia
Clear Cell Sarcoma   Soft Tissue Sarcoma
CNS Lymphoma   Lymphoma Colon
                                    Cancer

Colon Cancer
Craniopharynglomas   Brain Tumors
Cutaneous T-Cell Lymphoma   Lymphoma

D
Dermatofibrrosarcoma Protuberans
Ductal Carcinoma-invasive Ductal
Carcinoma ohm Situ (DCI*S)
Non-invasive
Soft Tissue Sarcoma Breaist Cancer
Breast Cancer

E

Endometrial Cancer
Ependymoma
Epithelioid Sarcoma
Esophageal Cancer
Extraskeletal Chondrosarcoma
Eye Melanoma
Uteri n/Endometrial Cancer Brain
Tumors
Soft Tissue Sarcoma
Esopjageal Cancer
Soft Tissue Sarcoma
ampma

F

Brain Tumors
Soft Tissue Sarcoma
Thyroid Cancer

Fibruilaryiary Astrocytoma
Fibrosarcoma
Follicular Carcinoma of the thyroid

G

Galbladder Cancer   Galbladder Cancer
Gastric (Stomach) Cancer   Stomach Cancer
Gastrointestinal Stromal Tumor (GIST)
Soft Tissue Sarcoma
Germ Cell Ovarian   Cancer
Germ Cell Testicular   Testicular Cancer

Germ Cell Tumor, Mixed Germ cell Tumors	Brain Tumors
Gestational Trophoblastic tumor (GTD) Gestational	Trophoblastic Disease
Glioblastoma Multiformae	Brain Tumors
Glioma/Astrocytoma	Brain Tumors
Glioma/Astrocytoma Granular	Brain Tumors
Cell Myoblastoma	Soft Tissue Sarcoma

H

Hairy Cell Leukemia	Head and Neck Cancers
Head and Neck Can Cancers	
Hemangiosarcoma	Soft Tissue Sarcoma
Hepatoceliular	Liver Cancer
Hodgkin's Disease	Hodgkin's disease
Hurthle Cell Carcinoma of the Thyroid	Thyroid
Hypopharyngeal Cancer	Head and Neck Cancer

I

Inflammatory Breast Intracular Melanoma Islet Cell Carcinoma (Endocrine Pancreas) Pancreatic Cancer	Cancer

K

Kaposi's Sarcoma	AIDS - related Cancer

Kidney (Renal Cell) Cancer	Kidney Cancer

L

Laryngeal Cancer	Head and Neck Cancer
Leiomyosarcoma	Soft Tissue Sarcoma
Leukemia	
Lip and Oral Cavity Cancer	Head and Neck Cancer
Liposarcoma	Soft Tissue Sarcoma
Liver Cancer, Adult Primary	Liver Cancer
Liver Cancer Metastatic (Secondary) Metastatic Cancer	
Lobular Carcinoma - Invasive	Breast Cancer
Lobular Carcinoma in Situ ((LCIS) (Noninvasive	Breast Cancer
Lung Cancer	Lung Cancer
Lymphangiosarcoma	Soft Tissue Sarcoma
Lymphoma	Lymphoma

M

Male Breast Cancer Malignant Fibrous Histocytoma	(MFH) Soft Tissue
MalignantHemangiopericytoma	
Malignant Mesenohymoma	
Malignant Mesothelioma	
Malignant Peripheral Nerve Sheath Tumor	
Malignant Schwannoma	
Malignant Thymoma	

Modularly Carcinoma of the Thyroid

Melanoma

Meningiomas

Mesenchymoma

Mesothelioma

Merkel Cell Carcinoma

Metastatic Cancer

Metastatic Squamous/Plasma Cell

Neoplasm

Myelodysplastic Syndrome

Myeloproliferative Disorders

Male Breast Cancer Sarcoma or

Osteosarcoma

Soft Tissue Sarcoma

Soft Tissue Sarcoma Mesothelioma

Soft Tissue Sarcoma

Soft Tissue Sarcoma Thymoma

Thyroid Cancer

Melanoma

Brain Tumors

Soft Tissue Sarcoma

Mesothelioma

Merkel Cell Carcinoma Metastatic

Cancer Multiple Myeloma

Other Blood Cancers Other Blood

Cancers

N
Nasopharyngeal Cancer

Neurofibrosarcoma

Nipple (Paget's Disease of the Brest)
Breast Cancer
Non-Hodgkin's Lymphoma (NHL)
Head and Neck Cancer
Soft Tissue Sarcoma
Non-Hodgkin's lymphoma
Non -Small Cell Lung   Non Lung Cancer

O
Oligodendrolioma Oropharyngeal
Canmcer Osteosarcoma
Ovarian Epithelial Cancer Ovarian
Germ Cell Tumor
Brain Tumors
Head and Neck Cancer Osteosarcoma
Ovarian Cancer
Ovarian Cancer

P
Pancreatic Cancer
Papillary Carcinoma of the Thyroid
Parathyroid Cancer
Penile Cancer
Pergheral Neuroeclodermal Tumor s
Pilocytic Astrocytooma
Pineal Parenchymal Tumor
Pituitary Tumor Includes Pituitary
Adenoma
Primary Central Nervous System
Lymphoma (CNS) Lymphoma

Prostate Cancer
Pancreatic Cancer
Thyroid Cancer
Thyroid Cancer
Penile Cancer
Soft Tissue Sarcoma
Brain Tumors
Brain Tumors
Brain Tumors
Lymphoma.
Prostate Cancer

R

Rectal Cancer
Renal Pelvis and Ureter Cancer
Transitional Cell
Rectal Cancer
Renal Pelvis and Ureter Cancer

S

Salivary Gland Cancer Sarcoma
Schwannomas
Skin Cancer
Small Cell Lung
Small Intestine Cancer Soft Tissue
Sarcoma Stomach (Gastrio) Cancer
Synovial Sarcoma
Head and Neck Cancer Sarcomas
Brain Cancers Melanoma
Lung Cancer

Small Intestine Cancer Soft Tissue
Sarcoma Stomach Cancer
Soft Tissue Sarcoma

T

T-Cell Lymphoma, Cutaneous	Lymphoma
Testicular Cancer	Testicular Cancer
Thymoma	Thymoma
Thyroid Cancer	Thyroid Cancer

U

Ureter Cancer	Endometrial/ Uterine/Cancer
Uterine Cancer	Uterine Cancer
Utereine Sarcoma	Sarcoma of the Uterus

V

Vaginal Cancer	Vaginal Cancer
Visual Pathway and Hypothalimic Glioma	Brain Tumors
Vulvar Cancer	Vulvar Cancer

Chapter Five

To My recollection, I was somewhere between five and six years old when I first heard the word Cancer, or Eating Cancer, as my adult relatives called it.

Mr. Buddy Wray's mother had the Eating Cancer in her breast, and had come from Atlanta to live with her son, and his family on the farm where the air was supposed to be much fresher, and the homegrown foods were healthier for her kind of problem«

Our farm was butted up against the Wray farm in Southeast Georgia, and the news traveled fast that the sick woman was coming home to die, and had an incurable disease, that was catching (contagious).

Beside the fears everyone had, Miz Alameda, Buddy's wife had Mr. Buddy, and their older two boys build a shack away from the main house, out in the mud fields I thought, so the old lady could die out there. Just like the Bible stories of people with leprosy, who were isolated to an Island. I was too young to understand that the Wray's house was small, and they had five children. When the grandmother came to live with them, there really was no room for her privacy, without piling the family up uncomfortably.

There was only the narrow red dirt road to Buck-head, that separated our farm from the Wray property. Each time we harvested corn near that road, I'd look behind every stalk, or pine tree, expecting a ghostly semblance of the elderly Wray woman to leap out, and enshroud me with the Eating Cancer.

Although scared half out of my mind for about a full year, Miz old lady Wray died, and I lived through the frightful experience that my lack of education caused, and no one caught the Eating Cancer.

My second most horrifying experience with Cancer was in 1950, when I started to Nursing School. In those days, in the absence of more conventional treatment for Cancer, like Chemotherapy and other methods, the system used for external cancers was the use of worms (maggots) The thought of this horrifying treatment made me sick to my stomach.

During the later part of the fifties, I'd already been an LVN for a few years, working the Neurology ward at the hospital where I was employed. Since that floor had a section of rooms that was not used for patient's care, the administrators decided to open it for a trial unit for oncology patients.

Although I was a Neuro ward nurse, I could hear the patients on oncology crying out for relief of pain, and other discomforts. Their call lights were on forever, and no one answered their cries for help. Finally, I decided that I'd try to help them, since my work was caught up for a while. When I entered that room, the odor was so intense, I had to leave hurriedly to vomit. I was so humiliated, that I cried in shame.

For two days I tried to think of ways I could bare to help those suffering patients, and then the answer came . As I attended an older patient of mime, who had halitosis (Bad breath), he lit a Salem menthol cigarette, and his bad breath disappeared.

I didn't smoke, but I bought a pack of Salem, and I took an ashtray, lit up a cigarette and entered the cancer ward. I read their charts, and learned that most of them were on pain medication that an LVN could dispense. I gave them medication that they needed.

I bathed those four patients whose hospital gowns were sticking to their open sores. And I bandaged their ulcers after treating, and cleaning them. I dressed them in fresh clean gowns, and sprinkled baby powder on their backsides, and sheets. Before leaving, they had fresh water as well. ,And then I noticed that two of them had dozed off to sleep.

I slept well that night, knowing that I had given a small amount of dignity back to those hopeless, and helpless patients. I made a report to the administration, which included instructions for proper care, and that ward was attended well until it finally closed.

Listen to a person who remembers what having cancer in the days before extensive research. We've come a long way, and still have a way to go before we can rest assured that we've defeated the enemy, the crab. So pick up your clubs, and together we'll fight to rid our world of the evil that lurks in the name of CANCER!

THREE MAJOR CANCER FIGHTING WAYS A PATIENT CAN HELP THEMSELVES:

- EXERCISE: Many patients may have a disability that can prevent them from exercising strenuously, But there are ways that you can accomplish exercise by following the following steps:

    - Step # 1: Sit in a comfortable chair that cannot turn over. Look straight ahead, lean your head to the left as far as it will go, then lean it to the right the same way. Now put your chin on your chest, and lean it back as far as it will go. Do these exercises about five times each day.

    - Step 2: Fold your fingers of your right hand into your palm. Now place the outside of your hand against your right rib cage, now lean that arm without moving your hand as far to the front as possible, and then back as far as possible. Now try the left hand and arm, Repeat these exercises five times each day.

- Step 3: Fold the toes of your right foot down towards the soul of your foot, and raise that foot with the toes crimped up toward your leg. Do this five times each day, and rotate to the left foot.

- Step 4: Repeat the childhood ditty as you do this exercise. "Put your right leg out, now put your right leg in, put your right leg out, and shake it all about.

- Now do the hokey pokey by turning all around, that's what it's all about. Repeat this little fun game using the left leg.

- Step 5: While sitting, or lying on your back in bed, or floor, take a fairly heavy book, place it on your abdomen, and pull hard towards your back. Try pushing the book away with your abdomen muscles. This exercise; may be stressful for some heart, and lung patients, so do as many as you can without too much stress.

- Exercising the urinary track muscles should be done any time during the day, but preferably while sitting on your toilet, to prevent accidents. Squeeze tightly like preventing urine from passing. Now push down as though urinating. Do this five or more times each day.

USING A HEALTHY DIET BEFORE DURING, AND AFTER TREATMENT FOR CANCER.

According to the American Cancer Society, balancing your diet by eating mostly plant-based food may cut your cancer risk by one-third.

Experts believe now more than ever that you have the power to live a cancer free life by changing to eat a balanced diet, exercise diligently, and avoid smoking and drinking alcoholic beverages. You will be choosing a lifestyle for cancer prevention, up to 70 percent of all cancers.

NUTRITIONAL Blockbusters that fight cancer:

ANTIOXIDANTS: Fruit, vegetables, and other plant-based foods are powerful weapons in the war against cancer. They're loaded with antioxidants, natural chemicals that reinforce your own anti-cancer defenses, by fighting free radicals. Since free radicals invade your cells and create cancer, all antioxidants are essential ammo.

Many fruits and vegetables contain the big three—Vitamin C, E, AND BETA CAROTENE. Then some are fully armed with additional antioxidants like flavonoids. These compounds give color, flavor, and taste to plants.

Cruciferous Vegetables, also known as Bassline, This food group includes broccoli, cauliflower, cabbage, kale, bok choy, kohlrabi, rutabagas, turnips, and Brussels sprouts. They all contain phyrochemicals with long names like isothio-cyanattes, indoles, and gluacosiniolates. They seem to safe guard your DNA from cancer causing mutations, they might even stop the growth of tumors. You'll get the most cancer protection if you eat these vegetables raw, or only slightly cooked.

ONION, AND GARLIC: These fragrant bulbs vegetables called alliums, also include scallions and chives. Minced or crushing them to release their full anti-cancer power. And don't over-cook them. Following these steps and you'll benefit form their flavonoids and sulfur compounds, which get free radicals before they get you.

Citrus Fruits: Oranges, lemons, limes, and grapefruit. These flavorful fruits are a two- for-one deal against cancer. Their pulp and juice are loaded with vitamins C. This antioxidants might prevent more than eight different kinds of cancer in one swoop; cancer of the bladder, breast, cervix, colon, and rectum, esophagus, lung, pancreas, and stomach, plus citrus fruits have antioxidants called monomer peer in their peels. Shave off some of this fruit's outer skin-the zest -and add it to drinks or dishes for the benefit of these chemicals.

++ BERRIES According to the ASDA-ARS, Human Nutrition Research Center on aging, these little morsels pack one of the biggest antioxidants punches, National chemicals like anchocyanin and elegiac acid attacks cancer-causing pollutants. So eat strawberries, raspberries, blackberries, cranberries and blueberries, being careful of the quantity in each serving if you are diabetic.

++ GREEN LEAFS: More vegetables with big floppy leaves and a dark green color-like romaine lettuce, collards, beet leaves and spinach contain cariotenoids. These high-powered antioxidants take out toxins and free radicals before they can harm your cells. Cariotenoids are especially powerful against lung tumors.

So passive smokers take note-green leafiest. As well as carrots and sweet potatoes can be the protection you need from pollutants you inhale.

++ TOMATOES: Lycopene is an antioxidant that sets tomatoes and other red fruits apart. This carotenoid appears to protect against cancer of the colon, stomach, lungs, esophagus, prostrate, and throat. Get as much lycopene as possible by sautéing tomatoes in olive oil, or by eating red pasta sauces and pizza. Snacking on red grapefruits, guavas, and watermelon will lift your lycopene level.

HERBS AND SPICES: Use these cancer fighters instead of salt to zest up your meals. Basil. Rosemary, turmeric, ginger, and parsley all contain flavonoids and other compounds that send your antioxidant level extremely high. Fresh herbs are generally more potent cancer fighters than dried.

GREEN TEA. People who drink about 4 cups of green tea a day seem to get less cancer. In recent test-tube studies a compound called EGCG, a powerful antioxidant in tea inhibited an enzyme that cancer cells need in order to grew. The cancer cells that couldn't grow big enough to divide, self destroyed. I would take about 4 cups of green tea a day to get the blood level EGCG that inhibites cancer in the body. Black tea also contains EGCG, but at a much lower concentration.

MY PERSONAL TESTIMONY FOR GREEN TEA:

My cholesterol was 250, and my glucose level was high also, with the prednisone therapy. I decided to use my mother's recipe of cinnamon, green tea, and apple cider vinegar three times a day. After about three months, I learned that my cholesterol was 136, and my hemoglobin which has a normal range of 7.0. I had dropped to 7.6

The normal range for blood sugar is 7.0 every three months. My mother's advice had brought it down to a percentage within normal, despite taking prednisone, a drug that sends your test high every two hours. I also found that the COPD (Chronic Obstructive Pulmonary Disease) the grand daddy of asthma and emphysema, had calmed down.

My aged mother's recipe of cinnamon, green tea, and apple cider vinegar, had done the trick for three of my problems: High cholesterol, COPD, and high diabetic blood sugar.

There are dozens other foods that contain antioxidants to fight off cancer, or restore cells after cancer attacks. Don't forget green teas polyphenoils, or olive oils vitamin E, and there is the alpha and beta-carotene in carrots. Load up your grocery cart with antioxidants's power and start challenging cancer.

SELENIUM: This trace mineral is also an antioxidant, in that it protects your cells and tissues from oxidation. For nearly 30 years, scientist have believed low selenium levels lead to a greater risk of cancer. Selenium is different from other antioxidants however, because a normal diet of mostly un-processed foods easily provide the suggested 55 micrograms a day.

Dr. Mark A. Neilson, a professor and researcher at the Arizona Cancer research says: The National Prevention of Cancer (NPC) trials trippled the intake and suggests that higher levels of selenium may be necessary for cancer prevention." Until nutritionists conduct more research, though, no one can recommend the best, safest amount you should set. Experts warn selenium is a toxic material, which means too much of it, especially from supplements, is unsafe.

For now, Nelson's advice: "Eat a well balanced diet." Foods especially high in selenium include mushrooms, seafood, chicken, and wheat.

++FOLATE: Folate is an essential ingredient in making DNA. Without enough of this B vitamin, you could end up with broken chromosomes, one risk factor for cancer. No wonder, then a folate deficiency appears to increase the risk for cancers of the cervix, breast, and especially the colon and rectum.

++FIBER: Dr. Denis Burkett author of the book, EAT RIGHT - TO STAY HEALTHY, AND ENJOY LIFE, first stated over 20 years ago that fiber might prevent colorectal cancers. Which diets are rich in dietary fiber?

Burkett said, "the stools passed are usually large. If carcinogens (the substances which produces cancer) are diluted in a large volume of stool and also if they are discarded out of the bowel fairly quickly (as happens with fiber-rich diets) rather than hanging around, they will be less dangerous.

Choose foods rich in insoluble fiber, the kind that won't dissolve in water-brown rice, fruits beans, vegetables, wheat bran, and whole grains, these are also rich in nutrients, and photochemical making them complete anticancer packages.

++OMEGA-3: Your body needs two fatty acids that it can't make on its own-lanoline or omega-3 and linoleum are or Omega-6. They're called essentials nutrients, and you must get them from foods. But you must get them in correct amounts.

When one type of fatty acid drastically outnumbers the other, things can go haywire.

Most people get more than enough Omega-6 fatty acids from a typical diet loaded with vegetables oils, and not enough Omega-3s found in cold-water fish and other foods. Some experts believe this unbalance is linked to cancerous tumors. Too many omega -6 fatty acids may promote tumor growth, while getting more Omega-3 fatty acids could prevent, or even shrmk-tumors.

With the battle between the Omega-3 s and the Omega-6, every week eat at least two servings of salmon, tuna, mackerel, herring, or other omega-3-packed fish. Include flaxseed oil, walnuts, and green leafy vegetables in your diet to boost your good fat intake even more, and just as important-cut back on eggs, milk, processed grains, and anything that contains corn or soy oils.

Trim down on red meats, too. They're high in fats-omega-6s and saturated fats. According to the American Cancer Society, a high-fat diet increases your risk of colon, rectal, prostate, and endometrium (uterine lining) cancers.

Be aware when grilling meats, poultry or seafood. Grilling has been linked to the risk of breast, stomach and colorectal cancers, according to the Director of Nutritional Education at the American Institute for Cancer Research.

If you must grill, consider marinating meats for at least 40 minutes using acidic liquids like orange juice, wine or vinegar. All these contain antioxidants and combined, they help prevent the cancer causing compounds called heterocyhclic amines (HCAs) found during grilling. A good prevention is to soak meets in olive oil, and honey mix.

++ CURABILITY OF CERTAIN CANCERS WITH CHEMOTHERAPY

According to Oncologist Dr. Miguel P. Median of the Kaiser Foundation, there are two types of cancer that can be cured with chemotherapy: They are Hodgkin's, and cancer of the testicles (Testicular) in young males, in retrospect, he mentioned that Lymphoma low-grade might not respond to chemo, while Lymphoma high-grade could be curable.

Dr. Medina stated that new help is now available for some cervical cancers, in the form of a vaccine called GARDASIL. The vaccine is mainly given to young females and young women, age 9-26. It is covered by many healthcare plans, and only a doctor or health care professional can decide if Gardasil is right for you.

What exactly is Human Papilloma-virus? As explained by Dr. Median in his gentle, soft Spanish-accented voice, (HPV) is a common virus, according to the Centers for Disease Control. 20 million people in the United States had the virus in 2005.

"There are many different types of HPV, some causes no harm. Others can cause diseases of the genital areas. For most people the virus goes away on its own. When the virus does not go away, it can develop into cervical cancer, precancerous lesions, or genital warts, depending on the HPV type.

Cancer of the cervix is a serious disease that can be life threatening. This disease is caused by certain HPV types that can cause the cells in the lining of the cervix to change from normal to precancerous lesions. If these are not treated, they can turn cancerous.

Gardasil is the vaccine given for quadrivalent Human Papilloma-virus (types 6, 11, 16, and 18) Reconbendant Vaccine. Four types only. Gardasil is given in three doses injections

- First, at a date chosen by you and your health care provider.

- Second dose is two months after the first dose.

- Third dose is given six months after the first dose.

Dr. Medina reminds us that getting the vaccine does not mean that close and regular check-ups with your doctor are not strongly advised.

++Chlorella another good source of cancer prevention.

A GOOD SOURCE OF CANCER PREVENTION AND LATER TREATMENT AID, IS Tung Hai Chlorella. Developed, and medically researched far out shines the Sun Chlorella type.

Chlorella is a member of lukaryatic organism (true nucleus plant), which has been on earth since the Precancerous period, over 2 billion years ago. It is not a sexually reproducible plant, but unicellular, fresh water green alga, which reproduces itself so rapidly into four times in every 20 to24 hours.

Chlorella is so small with 3 to 8 micrometers in diameter that appeared before the public only in the end of the 19 centuries. At that time, chlorella was named after "chlora" which means green in French, and "ella" which means a small thing in Latin.

Even though discovered in China, the Japanese are the leading manufacturers.

CHAPTER SIX

In order for us to be healthy, we must be healthy at the most basic level, the cell. Our cells are being replaced constantly. The primary agents which accomplish this are called nucleic acid. Most notably RNA and DNA. A diet rich in RNA/DNA is essential for the body to effectively repair itself, and is therefore considered a key to long life and the prevention of disease. Tung Hai chlorella is one of the richest known sources of dietary nucleic acids.

Chlorella is 2 to 3 percent chlorophyll. That may not sound like much, but it is the highest percentage of any edible plant. Chlorophyll is an extremely effective tissue-cleansing agent, helpful in manufacturing a healthy digestive track.

Tung Hai Chlorella is very rich in iron which plays an important role in the formation of red blood cells, the body's oxygen supply vehicle. Tung Hai chlorella would be a valuable food supplement, even without the nutrients listed above. It contains over twenty vitamins and minerals, including large amounts of vitamin A (Beta Carotene) and

B 12. About 60% protein as well. It is also a good source of dietary fiber.

Chlorella has a secret weapon that scientist call Chlorella Growth Facts C. G. F. This nucleotide complex is the driving force of chlorella, enabling it to strengthen and support the body's natural functions. Of all the therapeutic foods nature has to offer, none has as strong a physiologically activating power as Chlorella.

Tung Hai Chlorella contains no fillers, binders of recipients, no sugar, yeast, wheat, soy, corn, milk or sodium, no artificial flavoring or coloring, or preservatives, nothing but chlorella, it is grown under tightly controlled conditions in fresh, pure subtropical waters, and is priced well below other major manufacturers.

What chlorella will do for you is directly related to what your body does for itself. Allow the various systems in your body, circulatory, digestive, immune, muscular, nervous, and others, to be strengthened and balanced through the use of chlorella. This reason is clear. Chlorella's high concentration of important nutrients, Chlorophyll, vitamin B 12, iron, Organic germaniurai, and especially nucleic acids (RNA/DNA) nucleic acids regulates the body's production and utilization of enzymes, protein and amino acids.

They are the key to your body's growth, and repair mechanisms. The real beauty of Tung Hai Chlorella is that it helps your body become what it was meant to be.

The human body is an incredibly efficient machine. Under normal circumstances, it is able to turn food into energy, eliminate toxins, repair itself and reproduce itself, but like any machine, if its systems are out of balance, it won't turn as well as it should. The problem for Americans is that we don't live under "Normal Circumstances", for diets have become unbalanced, whether from indulgence or the quest for convinces . Our environment has become saturated with more pollutants than our life bodies were designed to deal with

Our lifestyles exert stresses on us that would boggle the mind of a man living under normal circumstances There may not be much we can do about out environment or the stress in our lives, but our diets we can control. There are things we can do to restore dietary balances. And one of those things can amazingly help to restore balance to the system in our bodies that are affected by stress and environmental exposure.

That thing is TUNG HAICHLORELLA., the amazing algae. The keys to health can be found in chlorella. Polysaccharades were the first substances isolated from Chlorella extract and tested. Chlon A, as the JAPANESE Researchers, named it, produced amazing immune boosting and tumor fighting results,. When tested against severe immune suppressing agents Chlon A significantly prolonged the life of mice given lethal doses of an infectious virus.

hi a separate experiment, Chlon A exhibited tumor cell growth. Some researchers believe that Chlon A is actually a beta glucan. Beta Glucans are polysactrarides that are found in abundance in some of today's most fascinating, and powerful foods, including the healing mushroom Aganicus blazei as well as microalgeas, and Chlorella. Beta glucans have been shown to be potent stimulators of the immune system. It is believed that they trigger the release of powerful chemicals that activate immune cells called microphages', Microphages actually have a specific receptor site for beta glucans "sort of a lock and key" mechanism that activates these immune cells. It is suspected that beta glucans may be the key nutrients that empowers substances to act as biological response modifiers.

Dr. Mark Drucher M.D. wrote that we can achieve balance with Chlorella. One of the key concepts of health is that of balancing. Balancing refers to creating a state of equilibrium, where apposite forces are equal. There are many things that negatively affect health? Toxins, undernourshing foods, physical injuries and illness, as well as life's challenges and stress.

Of all these harmful contributors, Stress, be it emotional, mental or spiritual may as well be the most destructive negative influence on health there is. Stress harms the body in a multitude of ways. First of all, when the mind is preoccupied with stress it is less effective in controlling and balancing organs systems and their functions. Emotional stress produces an increase in stress hormones that slow digestion and raise heart rate, blood pressure and blood sugar as well as weakens the immune system, leaving the body in a vulnerable state.

Second, stress causes the body to require a much greater amount of nutrients that are already in short supply. As an example, tremendous amounts of the B vitamins known as the stress vitamins - are required. Without supplementation typically the supply would be insufficient.

Third: A body weakened by stress is even more vulnerable to the damaging effects of toxins. Chlorella not only helps the body and eliminates toxins, but also provides B vitamins minerals. Antioxidants and building blocks for repair, making the ideal choice for a body under stress.

While perfect health may not be possible, better balance is clearly the goal. Improving health through balance will give the body more energy, help avoid illnesses, and injury and even provide reserves to help the body deal with stress.

Studies have indicated that Chlorella can provide critical benefits for congenital cancer treatment. The goal of chemotherapy is to gradually decrease the number of cancer cells to the point of which the body's own immune responses can control further tumor growth. To accomplish this, chemotherapy targets cells that divide frequently like cancer cells. Ironically, it also destroys the very same defense the body depends upon to fight cancer. Once treatment is complete—(white blood cells).

Cancer treatment that suppresses the immune system can cause a serious and sometime life-threatening side effect called "leukopenin." Leukopenin is an abnormal drop in infection fighting white blood cells. Not only does leukopenia increase the risk of infection, it can also delay treatment.

The scheduled intervals between doses of chemotherapy is designed to maximize the effect on cancer cells while allowing normal healthy cells to recover. Treatment delays due to a dangerously low white blood cell count can impede progress against the disease.

Studies showed that mice treated with the chemotherapy drug 5-flluororaexil

(5-F U) experienced accelerated recovery of white blood cells in tone marrow when given a protrewin-carbohydrate complex isolated from chlorella. Throughout the study, the chlorella group had a greater white blood cell count, thus they experienced a much milder form of leucopoenia.

Complete recovery of white blood cells occurred as much or twenty percent faster in mice given this nutrient.

Neutrophills are white blood cells that are able to ingest ;and kill bacteria,. Patients undergoing cancer treatment have an increased risk of serious infection due to a low neutrophil count.

Mice treated with the chemotherapy drug cyclophosephamide had an accelerated recovery of neutrophils if given chlorella extract. The white blood cell count was one and a half of the control group.

THE IMMUNE SYSTEM, ACTS AS THE BODY'S MAW DEFENSE AGAINST CANCER, AND THE SPREAD OF TUMORS. According to information provided by the National Institute of Health and the National Cancer Institute, studies indicate that "cancer patients have a better prognosis when their tumors are infiltrated with many immune cells."

The initial transformation of a cell into a cancer causes a change in the cell's production of proteins called "Antigens." When an immune cell called a "Microphage" devours a tumor cell, it identifies the antigens of the enemy for all other immune cells. Any tumor cell that displays that specific antigen is then marked for destruction. Antigen research is perhaps one of the most promising venues for new cancer therapies.

In fact numerous biotechnology laboratories are a few years away from developing antigen-based cancer vaccines that may reduce or eliminate the spread of certain cancers.

By enhancing immunity, Chlorella may assist in controlling the growth and spread of tumors. Studies indicate that Chlorella may be most effective in enhancing activity of immune cells that control the spread of tumors to other sites in the body, rather than those that eliminate the initial tumors.

As astounding as that research sounds, it does not reduce the need for traditional treatments. In fact, Chlorella's assistance is strongest in combination with conventional treatments.

CHAPTER SEVEN

A New Cancer Breakthrough

The first and only natural therapy proven on 400 studies (on people, not mice) Proven to boost survival odds up to a staggering 300%. In Japan, it's the best-selling, government-approved cancer medicine. Why then are Americans not researching into this simple mushroom contribution to the world?

I'm sure you're not aware that cancer just jumped ahead of heart disease as the #1 killer in Americans under age 85. Which makes it all the more tragic that Americans still don't know.

The shocking truth about today's best-proven natural cancer-fighter. Maybe some of you've heard that medicinal mushrooms can help you fight cancer. True—but there's a deadly catch.

The problems that dozens of different mushroom extracts are now being sold.   And many so-called "cutting edge" formulas are experimental long- shots.

Yet one under-hyped mushroom has been tested and proven hundreds of times—in studies on people

It's an inexpressive generic that most Americans never heard of. Yet the science behind it is so far ahead of better-known brand names.

Over 400 clinical studies on real people prove it works, so why are we sitting on it?

Have you ever heard of Coriolus Versicolor? Hardly anyone else had either, until the interviewer asked Dr. Mark Stengler why so many of his "incurable" cancer patients were now so fantastically healthy. In no uncertain terms, the doctor told them.

"If a loved one has cancer, you must tell them..."

The interviewers learned that a 10-year study proved that Coriolus Versicolor extract could even save the lives of late-stage lung cancer patients—more than tripling their survival rate.

Another fact they learned was that a 10-year study proved it can keep colorectal cancer patients cancer-free twice as long.

in China and Japan, it's not an alternative, but a mainstream therapy (they wrote) It's routinely prescribed for breast, stomach, colon and lung cancer patients. In Japan, it's one of the best-selling cancer medicines of any type. The proof that it works is so solid; both governments have even approved it as a drug!

Better still, you don't have to change your conventional therapy to get the benefits from this mushroom extract Just tell your oncologist you'd like to take it as a complementary treatment. Plus it is so safe and affordable; you could take it as a daily preventive.

Ironically, it grows wild in America-yet most Americans don't even know it exists, and tragically, even though a few well-meaning healers in our country are starting to recommend it, they're often prescribing the wrong form!

Even if you manage to find Corilus Versicolor supplements, chances are they're not the type that was used in the clinical studies. Many brands just consist of ground-up mushrooms— and simply grinding them up doesn't extract the medicine. Your supplement must be hot-water extracted or else you're not getting the benefit.

According to the interviewers, "It is easy to see why Dr. Mark Stengler's research is so important." "It's no accident why he knows secrets that have escaped so many other doctors. He's one of a relatively few naturopathic medicine specialist. His coveted Naturopathic Medical Doctor degree means that he trained for years in these subtle, yet lifesaving details that other doctors just don't know.

Dr. James F. Balch, M.D., wrote: "It's understandable why so many well-meaning experts got the facts wrong about these cancer-fighting mushrooms. Most alternative doctors had to teach themselves about natural medicine."

"Not only did Dr. Mark Stengler receive his doctorate from the prestigious National College of Naturopathic Medicine they made him an associate clinical professor!"

"The difference between a naturopathic medical doctor couldn't be more dramatic. In addition to getting the same basic training that all doctors receive, Dr. Mark Stengler received about 200 times more training in natural healing. He's a world-class, licensed expert in clinical nutrition, natural hormone replacement, homeopathic medicine, botanical medicine, psychology and many other branches of natural healing."

That's why Yale University and PBS TV asked for Dr. Mark Stengler when they sought to explore alternative medicine. And why so many of today's greatest M..D.s. are now saying that they can't think of a more skilled guide to natural healing than Dr. Stengler."

According to The Bottom Line/Natural Healing publication, a number of doctors praise Dr. Mark Stengler's research efforts.

"Known to millions worldwide as the Natural Physician, Dr Mark Stengler is acclaimed for combining the best of alternative and conventional medicine at his legendary clinic in La Jolla, California. And as you can see. both alternative and mainstream doctors are unsparing in praise for his revolutionary new breakthroughs."

"He's the one that other practitioners turn to for insight on difficult cases. Mark Stengler is the nation's leading natural doctor. Says –*Dr*. Steve Nenninger, N.D.

"Mark Stengler is the leader of the new wave of true healers— a highly trained physician who integrates the best of natural medicine with scientific research and real-life clinical experience." _Dr. Michael T. Murray, N.D.

"Mark Stengler is to be applauded not only for his healing work, but for his persistent exploration of the real frontiers of natural medicine, .a truly dedicated healer who harmonizes the best of the art and science of healing. _Dr. James F. Balch, M.D.

You may already know Dr. Mark Stengler from his dozens of TV appearances on FOX, ABC. and other networks, his weekly radio broadcasts, and his interviews, and articles in national magazine. In recent years, his discoveries have proven so spectacular that PBS Television spotlighted his genius in two breakthrough health documentaries.

Yale University sought his expertise for a cutting-edge study of complementary medicine. Top doctors and health professionals are rushing to learn his new techniques, and he's been invited to lecture in places as far-flung as Moscow, and Siberia. Many CEOs of Fortune 500 companies, and Film Stars, Famed Athletes, have traveled thousands of miles to be treated at Dr. Mark Stengler's famed clinic in La Jolla, California.

If you're wandering through the files of a Health Food store looking for Tung Hai Chlorella, according to Dr. Joyce Johnson, the amazing Chlorella, developed by the Sun Chlorella Corporation, saved her life. Doctors had told her to trade in her ballet shoes for a wheelchair but now she's dancing her toes off at age 72,

By taking her mother's advice to start studying ways to make herself well, she discovered the amazing Sun Chlorells, and started feeling better right away. Her problem had been toxins in the body. These toxins can lead to fatigue, inflammation, stiff joints, brain fog, weak defense system, and a host of other health worries.

Dr. Johnson wanted the world to know what had helped her, so she began speaking at conferences everywhere. She soon went back to school and became a nutritional doctor so she could help others solve their health problems naturally.

Now, at age 72, Dr. Johnson is still dancing ballet and having a ball.

It is extremely important to keep your natural defense system strong along with nucleotides in Sun Chlorella's high-powered stash of polysaccharide compounds called beta-glucans. People in Asia cultures have long used beta-glucans as beneficial foods in the form of mushrooms. Polysaccharides have an amazing ability to release powerful compounds in your body's own germ-stopping macrophage cells.

Two studies have shown some amazing results in one polysaccharides in chlorella were actually increasing the number of macrophage cells in the body—as well as reving up their activity. This meant a major defense boost to the study participants. Another study was even more impressive— it showed that clilorella's polysaccharides triggered the production of interferon, which you may know is the "gasoline" that powers your body's defense system "engine" that helps your body combat germs and more

And last, Sun Chlorella wakes up your body's natural army of protectors—called T-cells-with special proteins-carbohydrate complexes known as glycoproteins. These glycoproteins wake up the army and move them into action where your body needs them most.

Sun Chlorella also provides potent antioxidants and flavonoids to help you ward off free radicals that trigger health concerns and speed up the visible signs of the aging process. And it contains more beta-carotene and iron than carrots or even spinach to help improve your natural defense function.

Translated from all this medical language, that means Sun Chlorella can help you:

- Boost your natural defense system

- Keep your white blood cell counts at a healthy number to promote well-being

- Stimulate the activity and movement of your body's own supply of life-giving T-cells, which is critical for people with more advanced health concerns.

That's a whole lot of peace of mind when it comes to facing serious health problems. Nothing makes it easier to regain your health faster and keep you healthy for the long-run.

Together with your conventional treatment from your healthcare professional, you'll notice you just feel much better, stronger, and more protected-more than you will with any other natural supplement or whole food discovered.

Scientist, and patients alike know that with Sun Chlorella, you not only feel better physically, but mentally too.

So now you know there's no question that Sun Chlorella purifies and nourishes your body for whole health. But it also gives your brain vital nutrients it needs for better mental function and memory retention, too!

LISTED BLOW, ARE SOME OF THE REASONS THAT YOU CAN BECOME SICK, OR DEVELOP CANCER, AND THEY ARE THINGS THAT WE ARE IN CONTACT WITH EACH DAY

- 1. RESPIRATORY TOXINS Our air is filled with both indoor and outdoor pollutants that wreck havoc on our basic effort to breathe. Corrosives in air conditioning units can cause asthma and bronchitis. Dangerous ozone, carbon monoxide, pesticides, sulfur oxides and more have been linked to asthma and lung disease, along with headaches and fatigue.

- 2. WEIGHT GAIN TOXINS: To stay thin and fit, your cells need to be cleansed regularly. But when your cells are dragged down by toxins that lurk in fattening processed foods, they have a harder time tuning up your body. What results is a slower metabolism and "toxic weight gain" that's often blamed on ageing.

- 3. Fatigue toxins. Shocking amounts of heavy metals found in our water sources have been linked to fatigue, as well as to other health problems—all of which make us feel even more run-down and tired! Even your favorite cologne can cause fatigue due to a main ingredient called toluene, which can trigger headaches, asthma, seizures, birth defects and even cancer!

- 4. HIGH CHOLESTEROL LEVELS, BLOOD PRESSURE LEVELS & CIRCULATION TOXINS: pollutants from radiation, fried foods and processed foods can unleash an army of free radicals on your system and trigger dangerous LDL CHOLESTETROL LEVELS. Lead in drinking water has been linked to 680,000 cases of high blood pressure. Paints and solvents used in new construction of homes and offices are loaded with chemicals and gasses that can damage your heart, liver, and even your central nervous system without you knowing it until it's too late.

- 5. DIGESTIVE TOXINS: The PDA lists more than 2,800 food additives, many of which come from sources that are unnatural to our bodies. These can create a sluggish bowel with nasty symptoms such as abdominal pain, intense gas, constipation, cramps and diarrhea. The nutrient-stripped convenience foods we're now used to eating contain hormones, antibiotics, preservatives dyes, pesticides,, sulfur or tar-based additives, and more. These toxins float into the bloodstream and head straight to your weakest organs—so not only is your digestive system in peril, but your tissues, glands and blood supply suffer from toxic poisoning, too.

- 6. JOINT, MUSCLE & HEADACHE TOXINS: If you suffer from any type of discomfort, you should be aware that chemical irritations may be the root cause of your pain. Nerves are irritated by a host of environmental toxins, such as cigarette smoke, prescription drug use and even microscopic allergens in the air and water. All of these cause a chain reaction that often leads to inflammation and migraines.

- 7. NATURAL DEFENSE SYSTERM TOXINS: Something as innocent *as* the "silver" dental fillings you received as a child quietly release mercury, tin, copper and zinc into your body and drag down your immune: system. Breast Cancer has been attributed to pesticides in foods. Even worse, more than 10,000 bladder and rectal cancer cases each year can be attributed to trihalornethanes found in tainted water supplies.

- 8. Doctors across the country agree that the best way to get healthy is to GET RID OF THE TOXINS! Nothing detoxifies your system better than the breakthrough discovery of Sun Chlorella.

HEY GUYS! A TESTIMONY FROM AN CANADIAN WHO IS 82.* "'I sleep well and I still have regular sex twice a week. I recommend Sun Chlorella products to anyone who want a better life. Try it, it's; wonderful to feel good."

TYPES OF CANCER TREATMENTS

What treatment is best for you? Which methods have proven to be most effective? Here you can find answers to your questions, plus learn about what to ask your physician, what's new in research, and what you can expect after treatment is over.

TREATMENT OPTIONS:

Surgery: Surgery is determined by your doctor, depending on the location, advancement, and type of cancer to be treated.

The doctor will surgically remove the cancerous tumor, lesion, or a part of the affected area, depending on how difficult it is to remove, or if some other organ may be affected by the removal.

Surgery increases the need for good nutrition. It may slow digestion, lessen the ability of the mouth, throat and stomach to work properly. Adequate nutrition helps wound healing and recovery.

Radiation Therapy: This is the use of radio -active X-ray to shrink the tumor, or kill the cancerous cells. As it damages cancer cells, it also may affect healthy cells and healthy parts of the body.

Chemotherapy: Chemotherapy is the use of drugs to kill cancerous cells. As it destroys cancer cells, it also may affect the digestive system and the desire or ability to eat.

Biological Therapy (Immunotherapy). As it stimulates your immune system to fight cancer cells, it can affect the desire or ability to eat.

Hormonal Therapy: Some types can increase appetite and change how the body handles fluids

SOME TREATMENT SIDE EFFECTS:

Treatment of head, neck, chest, or breast may cause:

- Dry mouth - Sugar free mints, or cough drops, and ice chips

- Sore mouth
  Use warm baking soda rinse, several times each day

- Sore throat

- Difficulty swallowing (dysphagia)

- Change in taste of food

- Dental Problems see your doctor

- Increased phlegm - a teaspoon of lemon juice

Treatment of stomach or pelvis may cause:

- Nausea and vomiting

- Diarrhea - Take Imodium. tabs as directed on carton

- Cramps, bloating

- Loss of appetite

- Constipation - Take stool softeners, and Fiber capsules as directed on carton.

- Sore mouth or throat –Rinse with warm baking soda mouth wash

- Weight gain, or loss - Stick to a healthy non- fat diet.

- Dry mouth - Rinse mouth with lemon juice, or vinegar mixed with water.

- Change in taste of food - Try eating more fresh fruits.

- Muscle aches, fatigue, fever - For fevers over 100 F, call your doctor.

- Fluid retention - Mild diuretics should help, call your doctor to obtain this medicine.

WARNING: According to research personnel's Statement in the U.S. Oncology News, ABVRAXAN for injectable Suspension (paclitaxel protein-based particles for injectable suspension) should be administered under the supervision of a physician experienced in the use of cancer chemotherapeutic agents. Appropriate management of complications is possible when adequate diagnostic and treatment facilities are readily available

ABRAXAN therapy should not be administered to patients with metastatic breast cancer who have baseline neutrophil counts of less than 1.500. cells/mm3. In order to monitor the occurrence of bone marrow suppression, primarily neutropenia, which may be severe and result in infection, it is recommended that frequent peripheral blood cell counts be performed on all patients receiving ABRAXANE.

IMPORTANT SAFETY INFORMATION

In the randomized metastatic breast cancer study, the most important adverse events included neutropenia (all cases 80%, severe 9%), anemia (all 33%, severe 1%), infections (24%,), sensory neuropathy symptoms 71%, severe 10%), nausea (any 10%, severe 3%), vomiting (any 18%, severe 4%), diarrhea (any 26%, severe < 1)J) myalgia/arthralgia (any 44%, severe 8%) and mycosis's (any 7%, severe< 1%)

Other adverse reactions included asthenia (any 47%, severe 8%) ocular/visual disturbances (any 18%, severe 1%), fluid retention (anylO%, severe 0%), alopecia (90%, hepatic dysfunction (elevation in bilirubin 7%, alkaline phosphates 36%, AST [SGOT] 39%), and renal dysfunction (any 11%, severe 1%) Thrombocytopenia *any 2%, severe <1%), hypersensitivity reactions (any 4%, severeO%), cardiovascular reactions (severe 3%) and injection site reactions (1%), were uncommon.

WARNINGS, PRECAUTIONS, AND CONTRAINDICTIONS

The use of ABRAXANE has not been studied in patients with hepatic or renal dysfunction. In the randomized controlled trial, patients were excluded for baseline serum bilarubin >15 mg/dl, or baseline serum creatinine > 2 mg/dl.

ABRAXANE can cause fetal harm when administered to a pregnant woman. Women of childbearing potential should be advised to avoid becoming pregnant while receiving treatment with ABRAXANE.

Men should be advised to not father a child while receiving treatment with ABVRAXANE.

ABRAXANE contains albumin (human), a derivative of "human blood

Caution should be exercised when administering ABRAXANE concomitantly with known substrates or inhibitors of CYP2C8, and CYP3A4,

It is recommended that frequent peripheral blood cell counts be performed on all patients receiving ABRAXANE Patients should not be retreated with subsequent cycles of ABRAXANE until neutrophils recover to a level > ImSOQ cells/mmS, and platelets recover to a level > 100,000 cells/mm3.

In the case of severe neutropenia (<500 cells/mm3 for 7 days or more), during a course of ABVRAXANE therapy, a dose reduction for subsequent courses is recommended.

Sensory neuropathy occurs frequently with ABVRAXANE The occurrence of grade 1 or 2 sensory neuropathy does not generally require dose modification. If grade3 sensory neuropathy develops, treatment should be withheld until resolution of grade 1 or 2 followed by a dose reduction for all subsequent courses of ABVRAXANE.

It is recommended that nursing be discontinued when receiving ABRAXANE therapy, Severe cardiovascular events possibly related to single-agent ABRAXANE occurred in approximately

3% of patients in the randomized trial. These events included chest pain, cardiac arrest, supraventricular tachycardia, edema, thrombosis, pulmonary thromboembolism, pulmonary embolism, and hypertension.

DESIGNED FOR PREFERENTIAL (TP) ACTIVATION IN THE TUMOR:

XELODA is indicated as a single agent for adjuvant treatment in patients with Dukes C colon cancer who have undergone complete resection of the primary tumor when treatment with flouropyrimidine therapy alone is preferred. XELODA was non inferior to 5-flujorouracil and leucobvorin (5-FU/LVFS). Although neither XELODA nor combination chemotherapy prolongs overall survival (OS) combination chemotherapy has been demonstrated to improve disease-free survival compared to 5-FU/LV. Physicians should consider these results when prescribing single-agent XELODA in the adjuvant treatment of Dukes' C colon cancer

XELODA is indicated as first-line treatment of patients with metastatic colorectal carcinoma when treatment with fiuoropytimidine therapy alone is preferred. Combination chemotherapy has shown a survival benefit compared to 5-FU/LV alone. A survival benefit over 5-FU/LV has not been demonstrated with XELODA momotherapy. Use of XELODA instead of 5-FU/LV in combinations has not been adequately studied to assure safety of preservation of the survival advantage

XELODA monotherapy is indicated for the treatment of patients with metastatic breast cancer resistant to both paclitaxel and anthracycline-containing chemotherapy regimen. or resistant to paclitaxei and for whom further **anthracyclirie** therapy is not indicted, eg, patients who have received cumulative doses of 400 mg/oi2 of **doxorubicin** or doxrubicin equiva3.en.ts. Resistance is defined as progressive disease **while** on treatment, with or without an **initial** response, or relapses within 6 months of completing treatment with an **anthracycline-containing** adjuvant regimen,

XELODA in combination, with, **docetaxal** is indicated for the **treatment** of patients with **metastatic** breast cancer after failure of prior **anthracycline-containing chemotherapy.**

WARNING

For patients receiving XELODA and warfarin **concomitantiy,** frequent monitoring of **INR** or **prothrombin** time (PT) is **recommended.** A clinically important drug interaction **between** XELODA and warfarin 'has **been** demonstrated. Altered coagulation parameters and/or bleeding and death have been repeatedly clinically significant increases in PT and INR have been observed within days to months after starting XELODA, *and* infrequently within one month of stopping XELODA. **These** events occurred in patients with and without liver metastases. Age greater than 60 and a diagnosis of cancer independently predispose patients to an increased risk **of coagulapathy.**

CONTRASINDICATIONS AND WARNINGS

XELODA. is **contraindicated in** patients who have known **hypersensitivity to capecitabine** or to any **of its** components **or** to **5-fluorouracil.** XELODA is contraindicated in patients with, known dihydropyrimidine dehydrogenase (DPD) deficiency, XELODA is contraindicated in patients with: Severe renal impairment. Patients with mild or moderate renal impairment at baseline should be carefully monitored for adverse events. Patients with moderate renal impairment at baseline require a reduced starting   XELODA can Induce diarrhea, sometimes severe. Patients with severe diarrhea should be: carefully monitored and given fluid and electrolyte replacement if they become dehydrated.

If an adverse event of grade 2, 3, or 4 occurs (eg, diarrhea), administration of XELODA should be immediately interrupted until the adverse event resolves or decreases In intensity grade1. Subsequent doses of XELODA may need to be decreased. Please consult XELODA prescribing information for recommended dose modifications.

Women of childbearing potential should be advised to avoid becoming pregnant while receiving treatment with XELODA. Men should use birth control while taking XELODA. Women should not nurse when receiving XELODA THERAPY

Now that we've learned much about cancer, its causes, symptoms, and possible treatment, I'd like to talk about the testimonies I received from neighbors, relatives, and friends, who've battled the fears of being inflicted with some kind of cancer.

First, I'd like to thank these people who've spoken so candidly about this problem that most of us face each day, with all the carcinogenic contaminants in the food we eat, the detergents, and soaps, or lotions we use, and, the water we drink, and the very air we breathe. Rotating our life styles, are the only hopes we have. Change your detergent, lotions, and food often.

I promised the people that I interviewed that I would not use their last names, so their privacy will remain free of inquisitive questions.

RUTH was a lovely senior citizen whose magnetic personality was seriously contagious. She was well liked by her neighbors, and friends, and a piano teacher, who spent much of her time crocheting, doing needlecrafts, and spoiling her seven grandchildren. But unaware to most everyone, she was deeply entrenched in turmoil.

She had spent much of her retirement life taking care of her elderly parents, and now she had to deal with a chronically ill husband, who seldom appreciated anything that was done for him .He had been afflicted with an incurable Pulmonary Fibro tic disease, and was told that he was soon to die.

Not only did her husband have a terminal lung disease:, but he was also an insulin dependant diabetic, who struggled daily with his blood sugar fluctuating out of control. He was a daily strain on poor Ruth, but she always felt that it was her responsibility to keep her husband happy as long as she could.

Sometimes, he took advantage of her good intentions, and made unusual demands on her, or often defied the doctors, and tried chores he was not capable of doing, and would fall, injuring himself, and having to be rushed to the emergency hospital by the paramedics.

With all that Ruth had to do, her pastor made unreasonable demands on her time to play the piano for Sunday services, weddings, and other extra programs. This additional stress had worn Ruth's nerves to a frazzle, and she came unglued when she discovered the lump in her breast a few months before her husband's death.

Her first thoughts were anger denial, and self-pity. How could this happen to her beautiful body, she said to herself. She would not allow the doctors to cut away a part of her lovely body. (Ruth had the snow white skin that could not retain a tan, and she was above three score and ten.) but she loved what God had given her, and she would not depart with it.

Her healthcare provider chose to remove the lump, and affected nodes, and treat her with Radiation. She had to put her husband in a care center for a few days during her surgery, and immediate after-care, he thought that she'd forgotten about him and accused her of neglect.

A few months later, Ruth's husband died, but she is still plagued with grief, and fear, for she is loosing her sight, from macular degeneration, and the accumulated stress is almost too much for her. Her children keep her busy visiting with them, and the grandchildren, and her neighbors rally to her aid, by taking her out twice every week to dinner, or on lengthy bus trips with the senior citizens group planned trips.

Ruth suffered more from fear, and nerves, than from the cancer, and its resultant treatment. She is still nervous, and has recently been cured from a full body rash. She had enough courage to resign from the demanding church requests, and seems to be recoiling fairly well. Pray for Ruth in your daily prayers, that she will keep the faith, and continue her recovery; she's into her second year, and doing well.

LIZ was a happy-go-lucky full blood Hungarian who was married to an old fashioned demanding Italian man who was 15 years her senior. Never the less, she loved to prepare her native dishes, or Italian dishes, and invite neighbors over to share in the mouthwatering delicacies. She is the mother of five children, and several grandchildren.

Even though Liz was not born in this country, it is rare to find a pureblood person in this Heinz 57 variety of mixed marriages in the United States. Liz spoiled her demanding husband. (As if an Italian man needs spoiling). She danced to his music, and bowed to his beck-and-calls.

Liz's husband was chronically ill. Beside the dangerous inoperable aneurysm that was attached to his heart valve, he had other problems that required weekly kidney dialysis as well.

When her husband's physical condition detieriated, Liz felt pain in one of her arms, and was diagnosed as having a blood clot. During the treatment for this clot in her upper arm, she discovered a lump near the nipple of one of her breasts. The mammogram, and biopsy revealed that the lump was malignant, and a lumpectomy was performed, including the removal of several lymph nodes that showed a trace of cancer cells.

Liz told several of her neighbors how terrified she was, and they rallied to her rescue with counseling, and cheering stories of how they'd survived the same ordeal.

As she struggled to maintain her sanity, and her strength, her husband's care became an almost obsessive demand on her, between the dizziness, nausea, pain, fear from the chemotherapy, and oral medication, her thoughts were of ending it all.

As her treatment, and hair loss became more bearable, her husband's aneurysm ruptured in the middle of the night, and she had to deal with the ear-shattering screams he made in his final moment of life, as well as dealing with a Funeral, and the loss of an income.

Liz's life is almost together after more than a year, and she is optimistic about her future, She has been declared cancer free for the breast cancer, but recently they found a microscopic spot on her lung. She was advised not to worry about this spot, since it is so small, they are sure it can be taken care of simply. Liz is looking forward to a cancer free life in the future, and she spends a lot of time enjoying her grandchildren.

JOHNNHY MAE was showering to ready herself for her third sister's funeral who had died from breast cancer. As she ran her soapy hand over her breast, she gasped with the discovery that she also had a large lump that was partially hidden in the fatty tissue beneath her arm.

The sadness that I saw her face at the funeral was not all grief for her sister, but a sadness bordering on panic and fear.

When I hugged her as we filed by the casket to view the remains of her sister, Johnnie Mae whispered to me: "Big Mama, I've got to talk to you before you leave."

I'm not related to Johnnie Mae, but was the manager of the department where we worked, and I was always able to settle disputes between co-workers by talking to them, and there-by gained the name of Mother Superior, or Big Mama,

When the funeral services were over, and during the Repast, I took Johnnie aside to talk, and her tearful outburst was: "Why Big Ma? What does God have against me?"

I tried to explain to her that God does not single anyone out to punish, nor does He hold grudges against anyone.

In the midst of her fears and confusions, she explained to me why she thought God had singled her out for punishment, and she unfolded her sad story:

"I've learned recently that my little sister's eight year old son was fathered by my husband, his business is folding up due to the money he's spending on his young Mistress. Four of my seven children are in prison, three of my sisters are now dead from breast cancer, and today when I was showering, I discovered a large lump in one of my breasts.

Johnnie took my advice about seeing a doctor immediately, and having a counseling session with her pastor, but she'd not found the lump in time, and the cancer had metastasized, spreading to various sites throughout her body including the brain.

I visited her a few days before she died, and she had kept her faith in God, for she said to me: with a smile on her face: "What a mighty God we serve!"

VICKY was a lovely Irish senior divorcee, who had just become engaged to a wonderful man with means. After being alone for 20 years, we all thought she deserved a better life.

Before the wedding, Vicky decided that she should have a complete physical examination, and it was a good thing that she did, for the doctor found the beginning of cancer of the pelvis. She was treated for several months and was deemed to be cancer free. But the wedding was postponed indefinately. Vicky was afraid that at her age, the cancer could come back.

She still remains good friends with her proposed husband, even though there was no marriage and they travel together, and are having a wonderful time together.

BEVERLY came to our monthly Christian Writer's Critique session, and announced that she'd just beer diagnosed with Pancreatic cancer, and since most patients with this cancer usually died quickly, she wanted to say goodbye to her friends.

She did not appear to be afraid, but sad that she would not be able to complete the goals she had established for herself.

We all gathered around Bev. laid our hands on her and prayed individually, reminding God of the promise. He'd made to us if we believed, and obeyed. Beverly left the critique session that day, and for more than a year, we were not able to reach her by her E-mail address, or the phone number we had in our files.

Naturally, we believed the worse had happened to her, and her family had not notified us. About six months ago, Beverly rejoined our critique group, declaring that she had been healed, and the cancer is no longer in her body. Kudos to God, faith, prayer, and her healthcare providers who treated her.

John was a very spiritual man, he taught Bible lessons, and was a Deacon at his church. Everyone respected him to the highest, and sometimes, his minister would ask John to tell him where certain scripture was found.

John didn't smoke, or drink, and he ate mostly plain old fashion country foods, and he spoiled his wife of fifty years like every woman wishes she could be spoiled. They were the parents of three grown children, and a number of very successful grandchildren. He prayed with his family, vacationed with them, and escorted them wherever they wanted to go.

One sad day, as they visited my home, John's wife told *me* that she had some film she wanted me to view, and she showed me the results of John's colonoscopy, that most of us have every two to four years.

The photos showed two fairly large liaisons in the descending colon, and I tried to hold a straight face, but they looked me in my eyes for answers, and said: "It's not good is it?"

After a brief silence, and pondering what I should say, I thought that the only answer I could give was the truth. They knew that I was an ex-nurse, and would recognize a malignant lesion. So, I told them what they suspected, but advised them to get to their doctor right away with those photos.

The couple went for advise right away, but learned that John needed open heart surgery before he could have the colonectomy. (catch 22) During his preparation for the heart stabilizing surgery, his electrolytes dropped drastically, and he developed an infection. He fought valiantly, but each day of the month that he was hospitalized, his condition worsened.

John's wife and daughters sat by his bedside daily begging him to hold on, and not leave them. He fought restlessly trying to hang on for his family's sake, and he suffered terribly.

One day as I visited John at the hospital, his wife, and daughter cornered me and prodded me to tell them what chances I thought John had? My answer to them was a harsh, and stern one, as I told them in no uncertain terms: "Stop being spoiled brats, and let that man go home to Jesus to rest. Go in there, when he is awake, and assure him that he has done a good job with your maturity, and you can make it alone."

Two hours after John's family made the declaration to him that they would be all right, and he could go home to rest, John died peacefully, arid had stopped fighting to stay around to protect his family.

Each time Johns widow calls me, she praised me for helping them make the decision that they should've made long before the man suffered so much. She has become quite a managing woman for someone, who had to take charge in her seventies, and she is doing a good job It is good to see that she is paying bills, ordering workman to do repairs on her home getting car repairs and taking cruises without her husband.

Yeah for the truth!

VERNON was a fairly young engineer, with a wife and two very young children. They were happy with the gifts that God had given them, but before they got married, they had talked about having a large family, and they bought a large older house with a guesthouse in back in preparation for the children they had planned to have.

One day, when he was showering, he noticed that one side of his testicles seemed to be swollen. His immediate fears were of cancer. He didn't want to alarm his young wife so he went immediately for medical advice. The doctor told him that he could not find any reason for alarm, and gave him medication to shrink the swelling. After the medicine was gone, the testicle had become larger instead of shrinking.

Vern was then introduced to a surgeon, who felt that the; problem was serious, and he scheduled surgery immediately. The surgery was performed the next day, and the biopsy showed that the swelling was caused by a malignancy.

Vern solicited the prayers of his entire family, but his worse fears were that he'd not be able to father another child, and his plans to have a large family had just been taken away from him.

His doctor told him that his prognosis was good providing that he'd follow their instructions to the letter; otherwise he could die, if the cancer was allowed to spared. He had to take medication as instructed, and regular blood test. One time each year.

Vern's family, and prayer warriors continued praying for him, and today he is the father of another beautiful daughter who is ten years old.

Vern, his wife, older daughter, and son including his miracle daughter are happily looking forward to many years of cancer-free happiness, with lots of love from the family, and friends.

ROBERTA stated that in the spring of 1996,she had an annual mammogram. She had a sore spot in her left breast. The doctor said that it was like a thickening of the tissue.

The mammogram did not show a lump either, so they gave her an Ultra-sound in that area and they did not find a lump. They also told her that cancer is not painful, or sore in it's early stages. They told her it was fine and to come back in a year. The next year, they found the sore lump in the mammogram. She also had an Ultra-sound, and they told her it was malignant. Roberta says that regardless what they say, cancer lumps can hurt.

The surgeons removed the lump for a biopsy three weeks before her youngest daughter had a big wedding. Roberta was doing the reception for 350 guests, as well as making 6 bridesmaid's gowns. The results of the test show that Roberta had a rare form of "Poorly differentiated Edema Carcinoma. Which has a mass in the upper body, and sends out feelers throughout the body with new cancer.

Roberta worked like a trooper, preparing the reception and finished the last dress the night before the wedding. She scheduled another test for brain cancer the day after the wedding. And asked her daughter and her new husband to let her go alone as they would be on their honeymoon

At Seven a.m. Monday, that her daughter, and new husband were at Roberta's door, to take her for her test. They were wonderful. They went with her to every test that the doctor could think of, held her hand while she cried and made her laugh and laughed with her.

Roberta's sister, and her husband who lived in Sacramento, came to see her and prayed for her that the cancer would be gone. In July 1997, Roberta had surgery for the rest of the cancer cells in her arm and breast. They told her she did not have cancer in the lymph nodes. She was very thankful for that. They did not find any cancer in her body other than the one that they removed, and of course there was no mass too be found. God had healed her, she thought.

She then had chemotherapy—two types, every three weeks for 4 months. Her body did not handle this very well. The doctor told her she had every side effect that was listed for the medicine. She was so sick and weak she could barely walk. Her daughters were so good to help her. Her young daughter took time off work with permission from her supervisor (whose mother died earlier of cancer) and she or her husband went with Roberta almost every time.

When they could not be there, her other local daughter took her. She was too sick to eat the first two weeks, but the third week before treatment again, they would take her to dinner. She could not thank them enough for their help. There is another daughter who lives in Sacramento, two hours away, and they came to help Roberta on weekends when they could get away.

It is so nice to have a loving family, Roberta wrote in her testimony. When her family had to go home, that was not a good feeling, for she felt all alone. She vomited so often, she was afraid that she would choke when she was alone.

She developed esophagus infections, mouth infections, and sores on her lips, stomach disorders, headaches, weight gain, then a lack of appetite, and the inability to swallow, and it goes on and on, being repeated every three weeks. She had so many pills that one of her daughters made her a pill carton that helped so much.

The Lord was with her and she knew it, Roberta said. Often she would lie in bed and sing hymns quietly when she could not sleep. She loved the hymn "Leaning on the Everlasting Arm", "Count your blessings", and "Blessed Assurance Jesus is Mine." God put peace in her heart, and she knew that she was not going to die.

Her children were frightened but Roberta kept telling them she would make it through the storm. God would bring her through this, one day at a time One day as she sat alone, God gave her a scripture to read for comfort. It was Isaiah 43, starting in verse 1 that says: "I have called you by your name. You are mine. When you pass through the waters, I will be with you, and though the rivers, they shall not overflow you. When you walk through the fire, you shall not be burned, nor shall the flame scorch you. For I am the Lord your God."

There were times Roberta felt she was consumed by the illness of chemo side effects but she knew God would not allow it to overtake her because she believed in Him, and His goodness.

When she first had chemo, a few days later she ran a fever and had an infection in her arm and breast. They put her in the hospital for five days to give her antibiotics by IV, when she got home, her hair started falling out. She called her youngest daughter and asked her to come shave her head. She did and then took her to dinner wearing a hat for the first time. She could not wear wigs-they hurt her head and made the skin itch.

Every three weeks she could feel the hair that fell out alone, her neck collar line. She lost every hair on her body, including her eyelashes. When she finished treatment Including radiation, it grew back and came in blond and curly-like baby hair. In a couple of months it turned straight again but would not take color or a perm for many months. She had too many chemicals that remained in her body. Eventually, her hair 2 was back thicker but also whiter for the experience.

Next, she had radiation. That was easy after being so sick with Chemo. It only made her tired. After six weeks of this she started to blister and had the ugliest brownish gray colored blisters she had ever seen. She had to stop treatment for a few days to let the blisters heal, but then finished up the treatments.

When she left the Oncology Center after completing her full treatment they asked her to return for a visit with her family doctor, which she did. When he saw her he was surprised and said: "I never expected to see you' here again." When she asked why, he told her that with the type of cancer she had, she should have lived only two years at the most.

Roberta told the doctor that her family, friends and Internet of prayer warriors that her daughter had asked to pray for her, she believed God healed her. The doctor said: "You tell them that their prayers worked.

Roberta has been cancer-free for 10 years now and they are all still amazed.

NEW YORK MAGAZINE'S SURVIVOR MONOLOGUE:

In the issue of New York Magazine, published May 28, 2007, they interviewed 141 cancer patients. Of all those listed, 20% were breast Cancer victim, and 8% were colorectal.

The introduction to the article written by the interviewer of those 141 patients for the New York Magazine was so important to the information that I am trying to convey, that I thought you should read what that writer said.

"Elizabeth Edwards, Tony Snow, Fred Thompson, the sudden commonplaceness of cancer in the political landscape—and the extent to which *it* is discussed as something to live with, rather than to succumb to—illustrates the degree to which our attitudes about cancer have changed in the past few years, helped along by a vast and growing medical armamentarium. Two decades ago, cancer was a sentence with a period at the end. Now its rambling—discursive ending uncertain. What follows are stories that attempt to convey the blunt reality of "living with cancer" a phrase already ubiquitous and in danger of losing its specificity. No two cancers are alike, neither."

What a magnificent example of the truth about cancer, and it's wide spread epidemic. It is uncaring about where it strikes, whom it strikes, and what age level it tears down, or which family it destroys.

Thank you New York Magazine, for the article you published.

In the interviews that I had with numerous patients, they admitted that they put their faith in God, prayed daily for themselves, and others, as well as the medical personnel who performed their treatment, and follow-up, and many had others praying for them as well,

I recently read an article written by the research team at Duke University, declaring that they have proof that prayer heals. The article was surveyed in Durham North Carolina which read, "Numerous studies have confirmed that praying to a greater power relaxes lower levels of stress hormones increases levels of soothing nerve transmitters and reduces pain.

Duke University set out to discover that if patients could improve when others prayed for them. Their findings were that patients who were prayed for had drastically lower rates of complications, and the subjects never knew they were being prayed for.

Dr. Miguel P. Medina Oncologist at Kaiser's Antelope Valley facility confirms that those patients with a lower stress level, and optimistic out-look, seem to respond to their treatments better than those who are stressed. Be it prayer, or some other method of relaxing the patient.

Since most of the patients I interviewed said that they put their faith in God, and prayed daily, and had others praying for them, I'd like to add God's answers to the subject, as found in the Bible in the book of 2nd Chronicles, Chapter 7: which reads: "If My people who are called by My name shall humble themselves and pray, and seek My face, and turn from their wicked ways, then will I hear from heaven, and will forgive their sins, and will heal their land. AMEN!

Finally: Learn as much as you can about your body, dietary, and cancerous pollutants, You will never be able to avoid all of the pollutants, but do as much as you can. Seek a Dietician's help in planning a healthy diets for you to follow. Establish an exercise program that is best suited for you, and your age, or physical limitations.

Join a cancer care group, and discuss your concerns. Together with cancer researchers, our physicians, and other caregivers, we can send that CANCEROUS CRAB straight back to HELL, where it belongs!

GLOSSARY OF TERMS

ANOREXIA: Loss of appetite leading to severe weight loss.
ANTIEMETICS: Drugs used to control nausea, and vomiting.
ANTIOXIDANTS: Agent that prevents, or inhibits oxidation.

BIOLOGICAL THERAPY: (Immunotherapy) Treatment to stimulate, or restore the ability of the immune system to fight infections and disease. This treatment uses product from the body's natural defense system to destroy cancer cells.

BIOPSY: A small sample of tissue taken from a suspect site to determine if it is malignant, and the stage of malignancy I, II, HI, IV.

CALORIE: A MEASUREMENT OF THE ENERGY YOUR BODY GETS FROM FOOD. Your body needs calories as fuel to perform all of its functions such as breathing, circulating the blood, and physical activities. When you are sick, your body may need calories to fight fever and other problems.

CANCER: A name used to describe a broad group of disease, which have certain common characteristics. Most cells in the body grow and reproduce in an orderly manner, as dictated by the body's genetic information. A cancer cell does not follow the same genetic direction that Normal cells do.

CARCINOMA: Cancer of the cells known as epithelium cells.

CAT SCAN: Computerized Axial Tomography produces a three-dimensional view of the area suspected.

CELLS The smallest unit of tissue that makes up any Hiving thing. All cells have specialized structures, functions, and are able to reproduce.

CHEMOTHERAPY: The use of drugs to treat cancer.

CHLORELLA: A member of lukhyatic (true nucleus plant) which has been on earth since precancerous period. Over 2 billion years ago.

C.O.P.D: Chronic obstructive pulmonary disease. COLON: The large intestine.

DES DRUGS: Diethylstilbestrol, artificial estrogen taken during pregnancy to prevent miscarriage.

DIET: The things we eat and drink both liquid and solid.

DIGESTIVE TRACT; The parts of the body involved with eating digesting, and excreting food. It includes the mouth, esophagus stomach, and intestines.

DIEURETICS: Drugs that help the body get rid of water and salt.

DNA: deoxyribonucleic acid... Technique to isolate, reproduces, and label a portion of the genetic material.

DYSPHAGIA: Difficulty swallowing

EDEMA: The buildup of excess fluid within the tissues, such as in ankles, legs, arms, and abdomen.

ESOPHAGUS: Links the mouth to the stomach

FIBER: The part of plant foods that the body cannot digest. It helps to move food waste out of the body more quickly. Fiber is found in fruits, vegetables, dry beans and peas, nuts and seeds and breads and cereals. Fiber is not found in animal foods (meats, milk, eggs.)

FLAVONOIDS: The chemicals from which the natural color of many vegetables are derived.

FLAVOPROTEIN: One of a group of conjugates protein that constitute the yellow enzymes essential in cellular respiration.

FLUIDS: Liquids, things to drink.

HEAT THERAPY: Hypothermia is now being used experimentally. It may soon become a standard treatment since tumors are known to shrink when their temperature rises.

HARMONE THERAPY: Use of drugs that block hormones in the treatment of breast cancer, prostate, and other cancers. This therapy is used to prevent recurrence.

IMMUNOTHERAPY/BIOLOGICAL THERAPY: These are still in the experimental stage; it is to enable the patient's own body to produce substances that resist the growth of cancer.

INFECTION: When germs enter the body and produce disease the disease is called an infection. Infections can occur in any part of the body. They cause a fever and other problems depending on the site of the infection. When the body's natural defense system is strong, it can often fight the entering germs and prevent infections. Cancer treatment can waken the natural defense system, but healthy eating can help make it stronger.

IRON INFUSION: A compound from natures hydroxide (salt) used as a liquid introduced into the veins of anemic patients, or those who are iron deficient.

ISOHYPERORCYTOSIA: Condition in which the white blood cells are increased, but the proportions of the polymorphonucleas leukocytes remain stable.

LACTOSE: Lactose is a sugar found in milk and milk products.

LACTOSE INTOLERANCE: The inability to easily digest lactose. This may be inherited, or may occur after some types of surgery. Surgery related lactose intolerance may go away over time. Many stores carry special milk products that do not contain lactose.

LAETRJLE: An extract of apricot pits that some have proclaimed to be a cure for cancer.

LEUKEMIA: This is a disease of the bone marrow, the site of blood cell production. It is one example of a fluid cancer.

LYMPHOMA: This cancer attacks the lymph system, particularly the lymph nodes. MAMMOGRAM: X-ray of breast lumps.

MINERALS: Nutrients needed by the body in small amounts to help it function properly, and stay strong. Iron, calcium, potassium, and sodium are minerals.

NEUTROPENIA: Abnormally small number of neutrophil cells in the blood.

NUTRIENT: Chemical compounds (salts, protein, fat, carbohydrates, vitamins, minerals,) that makes up foods. These compounds are used in different ways by the bodies grow function and to stay alive.

NUTRITION: A three-part process that gives the body the nutrients it needs. FIRST, you eat or drink food. SECOND, the body breaks the food down into nutrients. THIRD, the nutrients travel through the blood stream to different parts of the body where they are used as "fuel" and for many other purposes, to give your body proper nutrition, you have to eat and drink enough of the food that contains key nutrients. OXIDATION: The process of a substance combining with oxygen.

PAP SMEAR: A test for early detection of cancer by collecting cells from the vaginal area to be tested in the lab. George Papanniculeaus a scientist developed the test.

PHYLOCHEMICALS: A class of helpful chemicals substances found in plants.

Many of these chemicals are thought to reduce your risk of cancer. PLATELETS: That part of the blood supply that controls clotting.

POLYMARPHONUCLEAR: A white blood cell that possesses a nucleus composed of two or more lobes or parts.

POTASSIUM: Mineral the body needs for fluid balance arid other essential functions. PROGNOSIS: Factor that predicts length of survival.

PROTEIN: One of the three nutrients that supply calories to the body, (the other two are fats and carbohydrates). The proteins we eat becomes a part of our muscles, bones, skin, and blood.

RADIATION THERAPY: Treatment with high-energy X-rays to treat disease such as cancer. External radiation therapy is the use of a machine to aim high-energy X-rays at the cancer. Internal radiation therapy is the placement of radioactive materials inside the body as close as possible to the cancer.

RNA: Ribo-Nuclear Acid

SARCOMA: Cancer of the bones, fat, and muscles tissues, and fluid.

SIGMOIDOSCOPE: A lighted tube inserted into the colon through the rectum, to look for problems.

SOFT DIET: A diet consisting of bland food, lower fat foods that you soften by soften by cooking, mashing, pureeing or blending.

SURGERY: An operation

THERMOGRAM: Detects growths by measuring body heat.

TISSUE: Groups or layers of cells that perform a specific function

TOTAL PARENTERAL NUTRITION: When a person receives needed nutrients through a needle in a vein.

TUMOR: This means simply a growth.

TUMOR NECROSIS FACTOR: A lymphokine produced by macrophages challenged by bacterial indotoxins. It has been shown to be lethal to tumor cells in vitro. It is considered to be virtually the same substance as Cachectin; Experimental studies of the effect of (INF) in human cancer therapy are underway.

PERSONAL KNOWLEDGE OF CANCER SURVIVORS

Name	CANCER TYPE	SURVIVAL RATE
1. Eula	Uterus	39 years
2. Eula	Breast	21 years
3. Eula	Colon	7 months
4. Malissie	Breast	21 years
5. Brenda	Breast	*20 years*
6. Sharon	Leg	25 years
7. Doris	Breast bilateral	7 years
8. Lynn	Breast	22 years
9. Ruth	Breast	2 Years
10. Roberta	Breast	6 Years
11. Edith	Breast Bilateral	15 Years
12. Jim	Prostate	3 Years
13. Ralph	Prostate	9 Years
14. Walt	Prostate	7 Years
15. Karen	Skin	21 Years
16. Vern	Testicle	12 Years
17. Velma	Breast	44 Years
18. Liz	Breast	1 Year
19. Nance	Breast	6 Years
20. Cheryl	Colon	12 Years
21. Leticia	Breast	7 Years
22. Dianne	Breast Bilateral	9 Years

NUMBER OF EACH TYPE, AND PERCENTAGE

BONE	BREAST	COLON	PROSTATE	SKIN	TESTICLE	UTERUS
1	13	2	3	1	1	1
1%	50%	1%	1%	1%	1%	1%

www.ingramcontent.com/pod-product-compliance
Lightning Source LLC
Chambersburg PA
CBHW020918290526
45784CB00002BA/603